IGFs In the Nervous System

Springer

Milano
Berlin
Heidelberg
New York
Barcelona
Budapest
Hong Kong
London
Paris
Santa Clara
Singapore
Tokyo

E. E. Müller (Ed)

IGFs
in the Nervous System

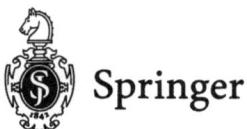

Springer

PROF. EUGENIO E. MÜLLER
Department of Medical Pharmacology
University of Milan
Via Vanvitelli, 32
20129 Milan, Italy

ISBN-13: 978-3-540-75042-0   e-ISBN-13: 978-88-470-2246-1
DOI: 10.1007/978-88-470-2246-1

IGFs in the nervous system : proceedings / Eugenio E. Müller, editor. p. cm. Proceedings of an international workshop held in Milan, Italy, May 16, 1997. Includes bibliographical references and index. ISBN-13: 978-3-540-75042-0   1. Somatomedin--Physiological effect--Congresses. 2. Insulin-like growth factor-binding protein--Congresses. 3. Nervous system--Physiology--Congresses. 4. Nervous system--Pathophysiology--Congresses. I. Müller, E. E. [DNLM: 1. Insulin-Like Growth Factor I--congresses. 2. Receptors, Insulin-Like-Growth Factor I--congresses. 3. Insulin-Like-Growth-Factor-Binding Proteins--congresses. WL 104 I24 1997] QP552.S65I34 1997 612.8' 042--dc21 DNLM/DLC for Library of Congress 97-41301 CIP

The use of general descriptive names, registered names, trademarks, etc., in this publication does not imply, even in the absence of a specific statement, that such names are exempt from the relevant protective laws and regulations and therefore free for general use.

Product liability: the publishers cannot guarantee the accuracy of any information about dosage and application contained in this book. In every individual case the user must check such information by consulting the relevant literature.

Cover design: Simona Colombo, Milano
Typesetting and layout: Graphostudio, Milano

SPIN 10572855

Preface

In the last decade, a mounting interest in the production, regulation, biological actions, pathophysiological involvement, and actual and potential therapeutic applications of the insulin-like growth factors (IGFs) has been registered. The important biological roles of these substances were first recognized upon their initial discovery as peripheral, circulating, growth hormone-dependent peptides. Continuing studies have revealed an increasing complexity in IGF function, highlighted by identification of the ubiquitous, autocrine/paracrine, growth-stimulating nature of these peptides, and by their presence from fetal life to senescence in a variety of tissues.

The new dimension of the roles and functions of IGFs, realized through seminal findings of the last few years, extends to the central and peripheral nervous systems (CNS and PNS). Recent discoveries include: localization of IGF peptides, binding proteins (IGFBPs), receptors and mRNAs in the brain, spinal cord and PNS; detection of IGF-I gene expression in stem cells during periods of rapid proliferation, as well as in selected neuronal cells at specific stages of development - especially during myelination and synaptogenesis; identification of IGFBP synthesis in the developing neural system as well as in adult brain; recognition of IGFs' neurotropic actions in sensory, sympathetic and motor neurons; and determination that IGFs are the most potent neurotropic factors in nerve and muscle.

These aspects of IGF research are up-dated and critically reviewed in *IGFs in the Nervous System* by a group of researchers credited for major advances in the field. In the first chapter of this volume, the need for suitable experimental models to study IGF function in the brain at molecular and cellular levels is addressed. Later chapters discuss the complex signaling pathways involved in the anti-apoptotic action of IGFs, the mechanisms underlying IGF-I's neurotropic effects, IGF-I's regulation of and its interaction with hippocampal function during age-related cognitive decline, and the mechanism(s) through which IGF-I exerts a dual role on target cerebellar cells - either protecting from apoptosis or up-regulating potentially harmful glutamate receptors.

Interesting topics related to the potential clinical uses of IGFs, discussed in subsequent chapters, include: the key role of IGF-I in regulating myelin production in the CNS and PNS by oligodendrocytes and Schwann cells, respectively; the beneficial effects of IGF-treatment on nerve and muscle functions in different animal models of motor neuron disease; the potential of IGF-I to rescue neuronal tissue in experimental models of brain hypoxia-ischemia; the rationale for use and effectiveness of IGF-I in neuromuscular diseases; and finally, preliminary reports on the potential therapeutic utility of IGF-I in devastating human neuromuscular disorders such as amyotrophic lateral sclerosis, post-polio syndrome, myotonic dystrophy and Duchenne dystrophy. Selected topics on the biological and behavioral effects of IGFs in the CNS and PNS are also discussed.

It is hoped that this volume may be of appealing interest not only to neurobiologists, pharmacologists, neurologists, and psychiatrists, but also to students of cell biology worldwide.

Cephalon, Inc. and Pharmacia-Upjohn are gratefully acknowledged for their generous financial support which made possible the publication of this volume.

Milan, December 1997   *Eugenio E. Müller*

Table of Contents

New Experimental Models for the Study of IGF and IGF-Binding
Protein Action in the Brain   1
M. HOLZENBERGER, E. GAY, S. DOUBLIER, M. BINOUX

The Insulin-like Growth Factor-I Receptor and the Central
Nervous System: Mechanisms Involved in the Prevention of Apoptosis   17
D. LE ROITH, M. PÁRRIZAS, V. A. BLAKESLEY

IGF-I in Neuronal Differentiation and Neuroprotection   28
K. A. SULLIVAN, B. KIM, J. W. RUSSELL, E. L. FELDMAN

Insulin-like Growth Factor I: Regulation and Interactions During Aging-Induced
Cognitive Decline and Impairment Within the Hippocampus   47
P. K. LUND, K. L. STENVERS, M. GALLAGHER

The Role of IGF-I in Cerebellar Granule Cell Survival and Terminal
Differentiation   60
P. CALISSANO, M. T. CIOTTI, C. GALLI, D. MERCANTI, L. DUS, N. CANU, C. BARBATO,
O. V. VITOLO, A. ATLANTE, S. GAGLIARDI

Regulation of Oligodendrocyte Development and CNS Myelination by IGF-I:
Prospects for Disease Therapy   72
F. A. MCMORRIS, G. S. VEMURI, É. BOYLE-WALSH, R. MEWAR, M. J. ENGLEKA, G. LESH

IGF-I and Glycosaminoglycans Improve Peripheral Nerve Regeneration and Motor
Neuron Survival in Models of Motor Neuron Disease   84
A. GORIO, L. VERGANI, M. LOSA, G. PEZZONI, L. CALVANO, C. FINCO, A. M. DI GIULIO,
A. TORSELLO, E. E. MULLER

The Potential of IGF-I as a Neuronal Rescue Agent   96
P. D. GLUCKMAN, C. E. WILLIAMS, J. GUAN, A. SCHEEPENS, R. ZHANG, V. RUSSO,
G. WERTHER

Neurobiology of rhIGF-I: Rationale for Use in Motor Neuron Disease 105
J. L. VAUGHT, P. C. CONTRERAS, M. MILLER, N. NEFF

rhIGF-I for the Treatment of Neuromuscular Disorders 115
V. SILANI, A. BRIOSCHI, A. SAMPIETRO, A. CIAMMOLA, A. PIZZUTI, G. SCARLATO

Insulin-like Growth Factor-I Effects on ADP-Ribosylation Processes and Interactions with Glucocorticoids during Maturation and Differentiation of Astroglial Cells in Primary Culture 127
R. AVOLA, V. SPINA PURRELLO, M. C. MORALE, F. GALLO, Z. FARINELLA, A. COSTA,
S. REALE, N. MARLETTA, N. RAGUSA, B. MARCHETTI

Anti Insulin-like Growth Factor I Antibodies Affect Locomotion and Passive Avoidance Performances in Sprague-Dawley Rats 135
D. SANTUCCI, M. LUONI, A. TORSELLO, I. BRANCHI, E. E. MÜLLER, E. ALLEVA

Neuroprotective Effect of GPE Pretreatment on Rat Hippocampal Organotypic Cultures Exposed to NMDA 145
L. CURATOLO, G. L. RAIMONDI, C. CACCIA, E. WONG, S. GATTI, C. POST

Expression of IGF-I and IGF-I Receptor mRNA in Sural Nerves of Diabetic Patients 151
M. GRANDIS, L. NOBBIO, G. L. MANCARDI, M. ABBRUZZESE, F. MARITATO, L. BANCHI,
A. SCHENONE

Subject Index 157

List of Contributors

ABBRUZZESE M., 151
ALLEVA E., 135
ATLANTE A., 60
AVOLA R., 127
BANCHI L., 151
BARBATO C., 60
BINOUX M., 1
BLAKESLEY V. A., 17
BOYLE-WALSH É., 72
BRANCHI I., 135
BRIOSCHI A., 115
CACCIA C., 145
CALISSANO P., 60
CALVANO L., 84
CANU N., 60
CIAMMOLA A., 115
CIOTTI M. T., 60
CONTRERAS P. C., 105
COSTA A., 127
CURATOLO L., 145
DI GIULIO A. M., 84
DOUBLIER S., 1
DUS L., 60
ENGLEKA M. J., 72
FARINELLA Z., 127
FELDMAN E. L., 28
FINCO C., 84
GAGLIARDI S., 60
GALLAGHER M., 47
GALLI C., 60
GALLO F., 127
GATTI S., 145
GAY E., 1

GLUCKMAN P. D., 96
GORIO A., 84
GRANDIS M., 151
GUAN J., 96
HOLZENBERGER M., 1
KIM B., 28
LE ROITH D., 17
LESH G., 72
LOSA M., 84
LUND P. K., 47
LUONI M., 135
MANCARDI G. L., 151
MARCHETTI B., 127
MARITATO F., 151
MARLETTA N., 127
MCMORRIS F. A., 72
MERCANTI D., 60
MEWAR R., 72
MILLER M., 105
MORALE M. C., 127
MÜLLER E. E., 84, 135
NEFF N., 105
NOBBIO L., 151
PÁRRIZAS M., 17
PEZZONI G., 84
PIZZUTI A., 115
POST C., 142
RAGUSA N., 127
RAIMONDI G. L., 145
REALE S., 127
RUSSELL J. W., 28
RUSSO V., 96
SAMPIETRO A., 115
SANTUCCI D., 135
SCARLATO G., 115
SCHEEPENS A., 96
SCHENONE A., 151
SILANI V., 115
SPINA PURRELLO V., 127
STENVERS K. L., 47
SULLIVAN K. A., 28
TORSELLO A., 84, 135
VAUGHT J. L., 105
VEMURI G. S., 72

List of Contributors

VERGANI L., 84
VITOLO O. V., 60
WERTHER G., 96
WILLIAMS C. E., 96
WONG E., 145
ZHANG R., 96

New Experimental Models for the Study of IGF and IGF-Binding Protein Action in the Brain

M. Holzenberger, E. Gay, S. Doublier, M. Binoux

Introduction

Insulin-like growth factors (IGF) I and II, along with their receptors and binding proteins form the *IGF system* which regulates important aspects of embryonic and postnatal growth in vertebrates [1]. The IGF system was initially described and studied in detail under its endocrine aspects. The recent discovery of important paracrine and autocrine IGF signalling has contributed substantially to understanding the complex biological actions of the IGFs. Expression of components of the IGF system in embryonic, postnatal and adult central nervous system (CNS) tissues, and their action on cultured neurones and glia have suggested a key role in development and maintenance of the brain [2-6].

Gene knockouts (KO) of IGF-I and its receptor caused severe growth-retardation and perinatal death in homozygous (-/-) animals and had strong effects on both CNS and extra-CNS tissues [7-9]. Some IGF-I-deficient mice which survived beyond the perinatal phase revealed defects in myelination and loss of specific neurones in the forebrain [10]. The IGF-II gene KO produced viable and fertile dwarf mice with impaired embryonic development, but with apparently unimpaired postnatal growth [11]. The cumulative phenotype of mice produced by conventional gene inactivation, however, does not allow clear differentiation between developmental or postnatal defects, and therefore is inadequate in explaining the roles of IGFs in adult animals. Studies using IGF and IGF-binding protein (IGFBP) transgenic (Tg) mice also revealed conspicuous effects of these growth factors on CNS development, especially on the myelination of new neurones [12, 13]. We expect that the conditional inactivation of IGF system components or their selective overexpression in adult animals would produce CNS-relevant phenotypes [14, 15].

Major advances in the study of cellular effects and molecular mechanisms of IGFs have been achieved through cell and organotypic culture experiments. Galli et al. [16] have shown that IGFs are implicated in the rescue of cerebellar granule neurones from cell death. The production of IGF-I in the Purkinje cells

INSERM U.142, Hôpital Saint-Antoine, 184 rue du Faubourg Saint-Antoine, F-75012 Paris, France

of the adult cerebellum [17, 18] suggests a role for large projection neurons in the local control of neuronal survival via this growth factor. Others have shown that IGFs have neuroprotective action, participate in the repair of nervous tissue and are implicated in regenerative processes in the brain [19-23]. It appears that IGFs regulate neuronal cell death through activation of the type 1 receptor (IGFR-1) and subsequent changes in apoptotic proteins in neurones [24]. IGF-I concentration is increased in the deafferented rat hippocampus, where its spatiotemporal regulation in response to brain lesions suggests a role in axon sprouting [25]. Enrichment of IGFR-1 on growth cones from differentiating neurones suggests a possible molecular mechanism for IGF-dependent dendritic growth and axogenesis [26]. Stimulation of IGFR-1 may regulate the assembly of microfilaments, enabling progression of the growth cone [27]. Clearly, more experimental models are needed to study IGF function in the brain on the cellular and molecular levels, particularly since IGF research promises to have significant impact on novel therapeutic strategies in the treatment of neurodegenerative diseases [28].

CNS-Relevant Effects of IGFs and IGFBPs In Vivo

Direct evidence for an important role of IGF-I in brain development came from the study of IGF-I-overexpressing transgenic mice [29]. IGF-I overexpression induced brain growth and axonal myelination through increases in cell size, cell number and myelin protein production (Table 1). The average adult body weight of IGF-I transgenic mice was up to 25% greater than that of wildtype animals,

Table 1. CNS phenotypes of IGF-I and IGFBP-1 transgenic mice

Gene	Mutation	Phenotype	Source
IGF-I	Tg overexpression from mMT promoter	Increased brain growth and myelination, number of oligodendrocytes, thickness of myelin sheaths, number of myelinated axons	[12, 29]
IGFBP-1	Tg overexpression from mMT promoter	Undermyelination, brain growth retardation	[12, 30]
IGFBP-1	Tg overexpression from PGK promoter	Brain growth retardation	[32]
IGF-I	Knockout	Brain growth retardation, undermyelination, loss of neurones in hippocampus and striatum	[10]

mMT, mouse metallothionein; *PGK*, phosphoglycerate kinase I

whereas the organ-specific weight increase reached 70% in the case of the brain. Interestingly, IGF-I levels in the CNS of normal mice were among the lowest levels measured in any tissue, and the IGF-I induction in the CNS of Tg overexpressing mice was also low compared to that in other tissues. Thus, relatively small changes in IGF levels may have strong effects on brain growth. IGFBP-1 overexpression, in contrast, caused significant undermyelination of the brain [12]. The dysmyelination resulted from both reduced myelin sheath-thickness and myelin protein gene expression. A correlation between transgene expression levels and growth of specific brain regions, possibly mediated by the stimulation of oligodendrocyte development and function, has been reported from a related Tg line of mice overexpressing IGFBP-1 in the brain [12, 30]. This model also revealed significant effects of IGF-I on the development of sensory pathways, possibly due to the regulation by IGF-I of neuronal survival and neuropil elaboration [31]. Another line of transgenic mice constitutively overexpressing IGFBP-1 revealed a similar phenotype with selective impairment of brain development [32].

Brains of two-month-old homozygous IGF-I KO mice were smaller than wildtype brains, hypomyelinated and had significantly reduced numbers of specific neurones in hippocampus and striatum [10]. Although not further discussed in the original paper, these mice showed a marked reduction in olfactory bulb size, possibly due to the intense neurogenesis and neuronal precursor migration normally found in this region. When olfactory bulb explants of late embryonic origin were treated in oculo with IGF antisera, they showed enhanced growth, an effect opposite to what would have been expected from transgenic experiments [33]. It is possible that in embryonic material IGF-I induces olfactory bulb (OB) neuronal maturation, resulting in an antiproliferative effect. However, the development of OB explants in vitro is probably different from the situation in situ since grafted bulbs are disconnected from afferent olfactory neurones and from the anterior migratory pathway [34, 35].

So far, the consequences of altered IGF and IGFBP expression in vivo have mainly been studied on morphological and molecular levels. Addressing a more complex biological function of the IGFs, Castro-Alamancos and Torres-Aleman [36] did site-specific injections of IGF-I-directed antisense oligonucleotides into the inferior olive and showed that conditioned learning of the eye blink reflex was specifically impaired. These interesting aspects of IGF action in the brain need to be confirmed and further explored in other experimental systems.

In humans, lack of IGF-I impairs normal development and function of the brain. Woods et al. [37] reported an adolescent with a homozygous deletion of the IGF-I gene showing mental retardation and defects in the sensory systems due to delayed intra-uterine and postnatal growth. Since the penetration of the IGF-I KO phenotype is variable in mice (only some homozygous mutants survive past the perinatal phase), one may suggest that null mutations of IGF-I in humans are not infrequent but do occur and in many cases are lethal during early embryonic life. The absence of IGF-I function in a particular individual may be partially compensated by the nature of the underlying chromosomal defect or the disposition of the IGF system regulation in humans.

Neuronal Replacement in the Adult CNS May Be Regulated by IGF Signalling

The olfactory bulb is one of the most IGF-sensitive areas of the developing and the mature vertebrate brain [3, 38-40]. The co-existence of two distinct types of adult neurogenesis in the OB makes it a good model for the study of neurotrophic factors (Fig. 1). First, sensory neurones in the olfactory epithelium are renewed during adult life. New neurones extend their axons until they reach the OB, where they form synapses with the neuronal network of the glomeruli [41]. Although the new neurones are formed outside the OB, the concomitant axogenesis and synaptogenesis take place in the OB. Second, neuronal precursor cells formed in the forebrain subventricular zones move rostrally through the anterior migratory pathway, and enter the olfactory bulb [34]. These precursors eventually differentiate into granule cell neurones. OB mitral cells, large relay neurones that receive input from olfactory neurones and project to higher centres in the vertebrate brain, express high levels of IGF-I during late embryonic life and, importantly, continue to do so during adult life [38]. The coincidence of highly localized adult neurogenesis and high level expression of a growth factor with a key role in CNS development raises

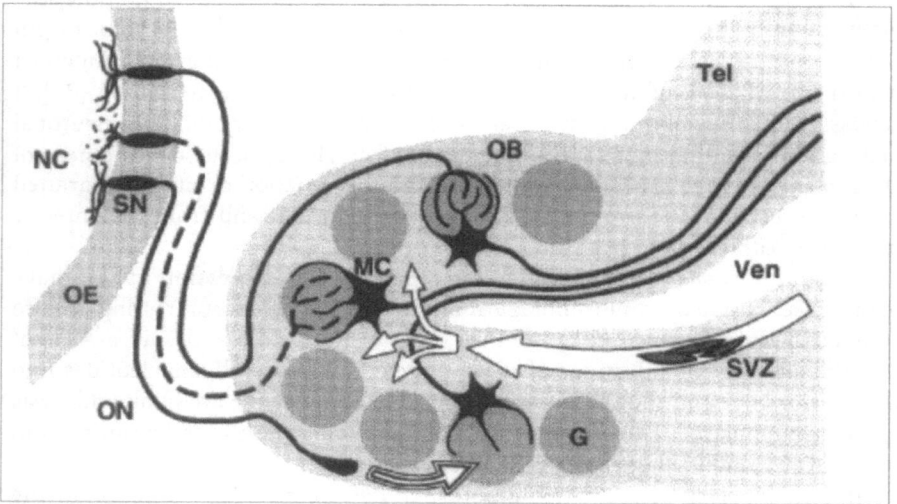

Fig. 1. Olfactory bulb cytoarchitecture. Sensory olfactory neurones (*SN*) residing in the olfactory epithelium (*OE*) project to the olfactory bulb (*OB*). They establish synaptic contacts with the olfactory bulb mitral cells (*MC*) and local interneurons, forming functional units termed olfactory glomeruli (*G*). The sensory neurones have a limited lifespan and undergo apoptosis. They are subsequently replaced by new neurones that grow their axons from the olfactory epithelium to the corresponding glomeruli in the OB (*double-contoured arrow*). Within the CNS, neuronal precursor cells are born in the subventricular zones (*SVZ*), enter the olfactory bulb through the anterior migratory pathway, and eventually differentiate into interneurons (*white arrows*). *NC*, nasal cavity; *ON*, olfactory nerve; *Tel*, telencephalon; *Ven*, lateral ventricle

the issue that IGF is directly implicated in the control of neuronal replacement in the CNS and may regulate aspects of plasticity necessary for neuronal replacement [42]. We found evidence of a similar role for IGF-I in non-mammalian species (Fig. 2). IGF-I produced by mitral cells may act on different target cells through multiple mechanisms: (a) signal to olfactory neurons like a classical target-derived neurotrophic factor [43], (b) stimulate axonal growth at the level of the growth cone [26, 27] and maximize the development of synaptic complexity, or (c) act as a paracrine and autocrine signal stabilizing the neurones in the vicinity of mitral cells during neuronal replacement and formation of new synaptic contacts.

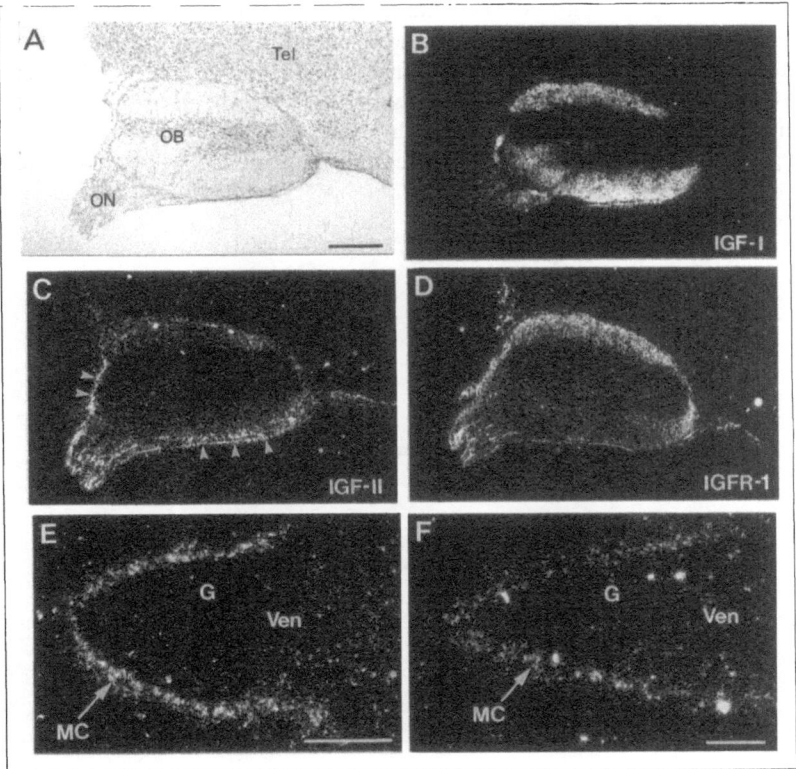

Fig. 2a-f. IGF-I expression in the adult olfactory bulb in non-mammalian vertebrate species. **a-d** Expression of IGF system components in the olfactory bulb of adult songbirds. **a** Anatomical details are given in a sagittal section of zebra finch olfactory bulb (*OB*). **b** Intense IGF-I signal was found over exterior cell layers of the olfactory bulb (darkfield micrograph of in situ hybridization). **c** IGF-II expression detected on an adjacent tissue section is mostly confined to the meningeal tissues surrounding the olfactory bulb (*arrowheads*). **d** Highly localized IGFR-1 expression indicates a possible up-regulation of IGF receptor turnover. **e, f** Darkfield images of chicken olfactory bulbs of 1-month-old (D30; E) and adult (D200; F) animals show high IGF-I mRNA levels and characteristic expression patterns detected by isotopic ISH. *Tel*, telencephalon; *ON*, olfactory nerve; *G*, granular cell layer; *MC*, mitral cells; *Ven*, ventricle. *Bars*, 100 µm

To further explore the hypothesis that IGFs exert a trophic function in adult neuronal replacement, we studied the expression of IGFs in the brain of two songbird species, canaries and zebra finches, that have become paradigmatic models in the study of adult neurogenesis [44-47]. In these birds, the CNS structures necessary for learning and reproduction of bird song comprise a series of forebrain nuclei, of which the high vocal center (HVC) and the robust nucleus of the archistriatum (RA) form part of the motorpathway for song production. HVC neurones project either to RA and or to a forebrain region termed area X. HVC receives afferences from another forebrain nucleus, the magnocellular nucleus of the anterior neostriatum (mMAN) (Fig. 3). Studies of tritiated thymidine incorporation and neuronal apoptosis have demonstrated that HVC receives large numbers of new neurones during adult life, and that this is part of an intense, HVC-specific process of neuronal replacement [48, 49]. This replacement concerns only one of the two subsets of HVC projection neurones (those which project to RA, but not those which project to area X) [50, 51]. Area X-projecting neurones and adjacent RA-projecting neurones form neuronal clusters.

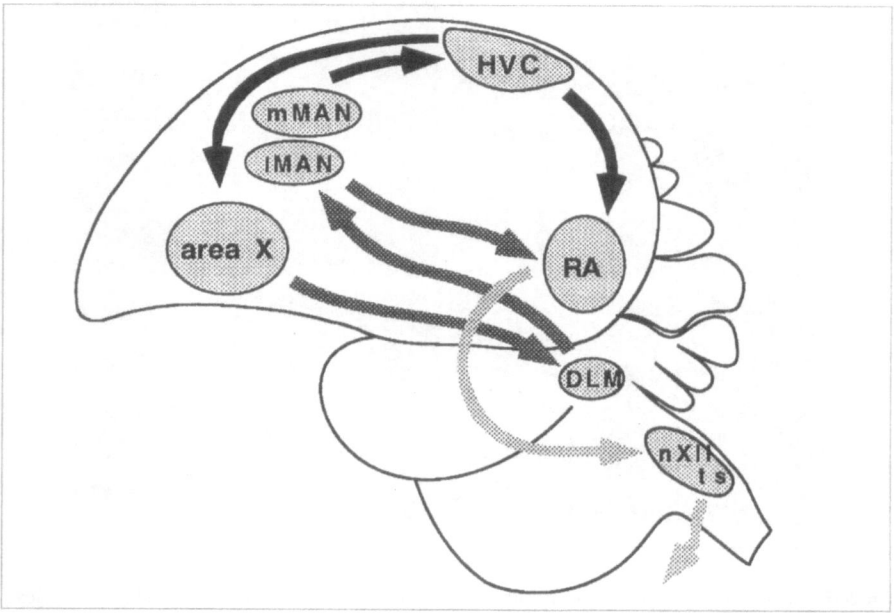

Fig. 3. Brain nuclei necessary for song learning and the neuronal projections between them. Two distinct neuronal populations have been identified in the high vocal centre (*HVC*). One projects to *Area X* and the other to the robust nucleus of the archistriatum (*RA*). HVC neurones receive afferences from the medial portion of the magnocellular nucleus of the anterior neostriatum (*mMAN*). Together with RA, the tracheosyringeal portion of the hypoglossal nucleus (*nXIIts*) forms part of the motorpathway that controls song production in the syrinx. Area X, the dorsolateral thalamic nucleus (*DLM*) and lateral MAN (*lMAN*) are important for the acquisition of learned song. HVC, RA and mMAN neurones express high levels of IGF-II mRNA (see Fig. 5)

HVC neurones receive afferents from mMAN (Fig. 4). Replacement of RA projection neurones in HVC causes cytoarchitectural changes not only within HVC, but certainly also downstream in RA, and possibly upstream in mMAN.

Using in situ hybridization (ISH) we found highly specific IGF-II mRNA expression in HVC, mMAN and (to a variable extent) in RA (Fig. 5). An IGF-II specific antibody revealed that the growth factor immunoreactivity itself was also enriched in HVC and mMAN [47]. Taken together our findings suggest that forebrain structures participating in the remodelling of neuronal circuitry due to neuronal replacement in HVC also express high levels of IGF-II. ISH and immunocytochemistry (ICC), in combination with neuronal tracer studies, revealed that non-replaceable (area X-projecting) neurones synthesized IGF-II mRNA, but that the IGF-II immunoreactivity was confined to RA-projecting neurones [47]. IGF-II immunoreactivity was located intracellularly in RA-projecting neurons in a perinuclear distribution. These findings suggest that IGF-II is produced and secreted by area X-projecting neurons, and taken up by RA-projecting neurons.

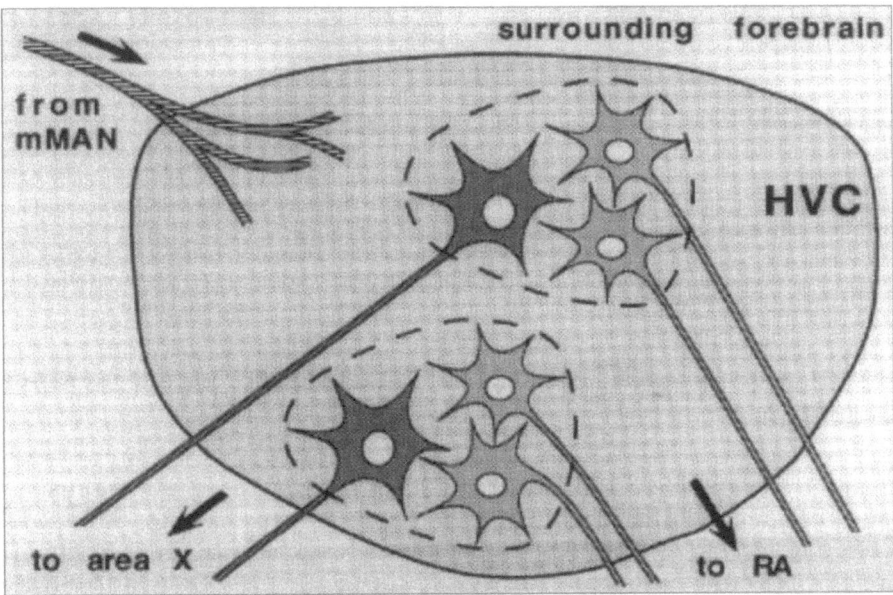

Fig. 4. Neuroarchitecture of the songbird HVC. RA- and Area X-projecting neurons often form cell clusters which could be the functional units of HVC's neuronal circuitry (*circles with dashed lines*). HVC neurons receive afferences from mMAN, but the exact neuronal connections within HVC are still unknown

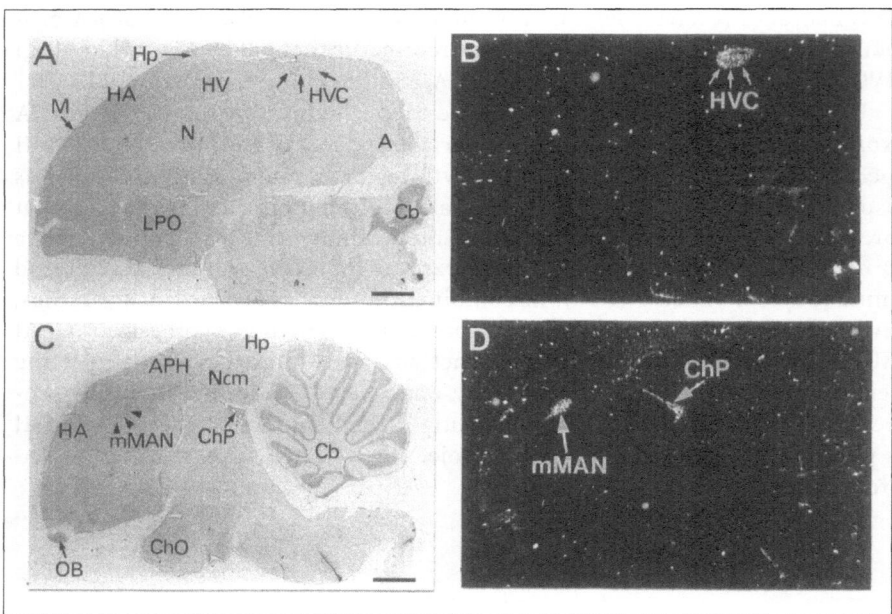

Fig. 5a-d. Specific IGF-II expression in songnuclei of adult canaries detected by radioisotopic ISH. **a, c** Parasaggital sections of canary brain through HVC (A) and mMAN (C). **b, d** Corresponding darkfield micrographs show intense expression of IGF-II in HVC, mMAN and choroid plexus, and conspicuous expression in hippocampus, parahippocampus, Purkinje cells and meninges. *A,* archistriatum; *APH,* area parahippocampalis; *OB,* olfactory bulb; *Cb,* cerebellum; *ChO,* chiasma opticum; *ChP,* choroid plexus; *HA,* hyperstriatum accessorium; *Hp,* hippocampus; *HV,* hyperstriatum ventrale; *LPO,* lobus parolfactorius; *M,* meninges; *N,* neostriatum; *Ncm,* caudomedial neostriatum. *Bars,* 1 mm

Regulation of Neuronal Plasticity and Survival Through Paracrine Growth Factor Signals

At any given time only a small fraction of RA-projecting cells in HVC is actually being replaced, while the majority remains stable. The fact that most of the RA-projecting cells do contain IGF-II immunoreactivity, and that the majority of Area X-projecting cells express IGF-II mRNA favour the view that IGF-II is implicated in the stabilization of neuronal structures, but that it does not directly control the dynamic process through which single neurones are eliminated (Fig. 6). This suggests an IGF action in the song nuclei comparable to the inhibition of apoptosis described in other systems [16, 52]. Speculating on the consequences of the neurogenetic events in HVC, this nucleus could be considered to be a hot spot of neuronal plasticity, where dendritic arborizations and synaptic contacts are remodelled at high rates, and where neurones that cannot adapt to changes in neuronal connectivity are not maintained. IGF-II could act as a neurotrophic substance that allows high degrees of plasticity, including the

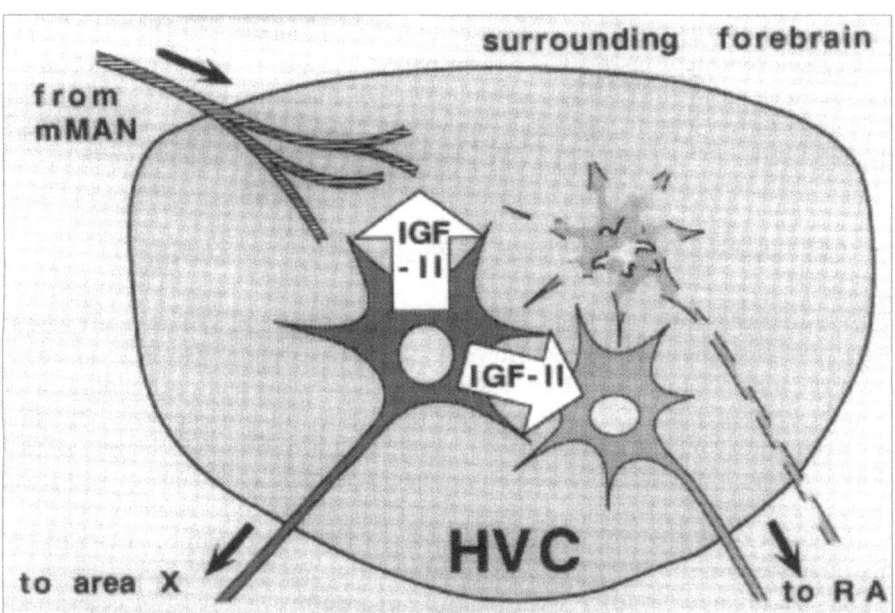

Fig. 6. Potential targets for the neurotrophic action of IGF-II produced by Area X-projecting HVC neurones. Some of the RA-projecting neurones are subject to neuronal apoptosis and are replaced (dashed outlines), while others are maintained. This replacement is likely to produce subsequent changes in synaptic contacts with neighbouring cells and afferent projections. IGF-II may be produced by Area X-projecting neurones to stabilize or rescue RA cells that are not to be replaced, and to create a trophic environment that allows rapid growth of new neurites and efficient neosynaptogenesis

complete replacement of neurones in defined areas of the CNS. Such an interpretation could also explain why in some other parts of the adult brain where neural plasticity is important but where neural replacement has not been described (e.g. Purkinje cells in the cerebellum), we do observe selective IGF expression by large projection neurones. Interestingly, the hippocampus and parahippocampus, other important sites of localized IGF-II expression in the brains of adult birds, also show high degrees of neuronal replacement [53, 54].

Intriguing questions remain: Why do HVC neurones express IGF-II and not IGF-I, while in all other species studied olfactory bulb mitral cells preferentially use IGF-I? What is the significance of constitutive IGF-II expression in the choroid plexus and the leptomeningeal cells? IGF-II, one of the major proteins produced by the epithelial cells of the choroid plexus [55], is secreted into the cerebrospinal fluid (CSF). It is plausible that plexus-derived IGF-II is available to many, if not all, CNS tissues. What is the functional difference between IGF-II supplied via para/autocrine or neuroendocrine pathways for cells in the CNS? The bioavailability of neuroendocrine IGF-II certainly depends on specific interactions with high affinity binding proteins (IGFBP-2 and -6) present in the

CSF [56, 57]. IGF-II synthesized and secreted locally may be targeted to immediately adjacent neurons or may act on nerve endings of afferent projections. Interactions with IGFBPs may result in selective effects on individual, adjacent cells; association with IGFBPs may impose a temporal regulation of IGF action on target cells.

The CNS Could be a Primary Target for Postnatally Expressed IGFs

The choroid plexus is a primary neuroendocrine source of IFG-II in all vertebrate species studied [47, 58, 59]. However, the precise role of IGF-II in the adult brain remains obscure. IGF-II knockout mice showed normal postnatal growth (which is essentially IGF-I-dependent), but they did not recover from the impaired embryonic development [7]. One possibility, although largely unexplored, is that IGF-I to some degree compensates for the absence of IGF-II in the CSF and the brain. Some of the questions, however, concerning endocrine, neuroendocrine and paracrine effects of IGF system components can be answered studying IGFBP Tg mice with different promoter characteristics.

We established Tg mice with hepato-specific overexpression of human IGFBP-1 (hIGFBP-I) under control of the alpha-1 antitrypsin promoter that allows localized transgene expression in the liver, site of physiological IGFBP-1 biosynthesis. We aimed to investigate the endocrine effects of IGFBP-1 overexpression, and to compare them with the results of overexpression obtained using the PGK- or mMT-promoters [12, 32]. Homozygous Tg mice produced hIGFBP-1 during late embryogenesis, in the perinatal period and throughout adult life. Two lines of these transgenic mice showed a phenotype of delayed, but proportionate somatic growth and impaired reproductive behaviour and fertility [60]. Failure to grow was significant in homozygotic overexpressing animals from the second week of postnatal life. Absolute brain weight was inferior to that of wildtype, but relative brain weight compared to total weight was increased. In the adult homozygous Tg animal average circulating hIGFBP-1 levels were moderately increased (14 ng/ml vs. 3 ng/ml in heterozygotes). Significant concentrations of IGFBP-1 (10% and 50% of the plasma levels) were found in the CSF of two homozygous Tg animals. IGF-I plasma levels in homozygotes with severe growth retardation were only 60% of normal values. We observed a dysregulation of blood glucose levels in hypo- and hyperglycemia tests that could be explained by an enlarged pool of IGFBP-1 in the general circulation. The most visible abnormality of the CNS in homozygous Tg mice was hydrocephalus, which was apparent in one-third of the cases. Brains of homozygous IGFBP-1-overexpressing mice displayed developmental defects (Table 2). The lateral ventricles of the brains were substantially enlarged; the corpus callosum showed general atrophia and degenerated fibre tracts could be seen at higher magnification. The hippocampus was compressed and shortened to roughly half the normal size. Most importantly, the cerebral cortex was thinner than that of normal mice and appeared disorganized, making the identifica-

Table 2. CNS phenotypes of homozygous and heterozygous transgenic mice with liver-specific overexpression of hIGFBP-1

CNS structure	Homozygous mice	Heterozygous mice
Cerebral cortex	Thin, disorganised cytoarchitecture, presence of pycnotic cells	Histologically normal stratification of cell layers
Hippocampus	Dentate gyrus shortened and compressed	No apparent abnormalities
Corpus callosum	Atrophia, degenerated fibre tracts	Thin, some degenerated fibre tracts
Cerebral ventricles	Important dilatation of lateral ventricles	Normal or slightly enlarged lateral ventricles
Cerebellum	No apparent abnormalities	No apparent abnormalities

tion of cortical cell layers difficult. Pycnotic figures were frequently seen. The cerebellum, however, showed no apparent abnormalities.

In this Tg mouse model, hepatic expression of IGF-I and IGFBP-1 is no longer co-regulated as it is in the wild-type animal. Northern analysis did not reveal ectopic expression of the hIGFBP-1 transgene in the brain. Diminished bioavailability of IGF-I through its sequestration by IGFBP-1 is a plausible explanation for most of the phenotypic changes observed in homozygous Tg animals. In particular, we propose that during development and postnatal growth, hIGFBP-1 of transgenic origin reduces the biologically active levels of both locally produced and circulating IGFs in the CNS, causing defects in neurone and axon formation. The insufficient development of neuronal networks may in turn cause enhanced cellular death in the cortical areas resulting in brains with atrophic fibre tracts (e.g. corpus callosum) and disorganized cerebral cortex. The fact that we detected hIGFBP-1 in the CSF of animals at an age when the blood brain barrier (BBB) is normally functional suggests that the BBB in our IGFBP-1 Tg animals may be deficient, a possibility that we are currently exploring.

Several of the major phenotypic traits of our IGFBP-1 Tg mouse are also typical of the postnatal survivors of the IGF-I KO mouse (brain growth retardation, reduced thickness of corpus callosum, strongly reduced size of the dentate gyrus, and loss of neurones in hippocampus and striatum [10]), suggesting that overexpression of IGFBP-1 mimics an IGF-I KO phenotype. Therefore, circulating IGFBP-1 is an effective inhibitor of the IGF-I action during brain development and maturation. The principal defects in CNS development due to perturbation of the IGF system could ultimately be attributed to the failure to establish sufficient contact between projection neurones and their respective target area neurones and to insufficient axonal myelination. This phenotype also confirms that IGFBPs act far from their site of synthesis and suggests that the biological effects of locally produced IGF can be inhibited by circulating IGFBP-1.

Development of a Mouse Model to Study IGF Action in the Adult Brain

It is clear that IGF signalling has important roles in the adult CNS [61]. What would be the direct consequences and specific phenotypic changes in a vertebrate model in which IGF signalling could be effectively suppressed at a given time during adult life or in a given tissue? Recent advances in the targeted manipulation of the mouse genome now provide alternatives to dominant negative approaches or antisense strategies for in vivo studies. Conditional gene inactivation using the *Cre-LoxP* recombination system allows investigators to shut off a gene of interest at a given point of development or during adult life by a molecular switch [62, 63]. We have designed and constructed a replacement vector for mutation of the IGFR-1 receptor gene following strategies developed by Rajewski and co-workers [64]. We have introduced the necessary *LoxP* mutation of the IGFR-1 gene into the genome of embryonic stem (ES) cells and we are in the process of passing the mutation into the germ line. The effective inducibility of such a conditional KO depends on the possibility to express sufficient amounts of the recombinase Cre in the target tissues upon administration of an exogenous substance. We are currently developing a *Cre*-transgene based on the tetracycline-inducible promoters developed by Bujard and co-workers [65, 66].

Conclusion

The songbird brain has been introduced as a model for the study of IGF action in the vertebrate brain. We have demonstrated that there might be a close link between neuronal replacement, plasticity and IGF ligand expression. The songsystem nuclei of canary and zebra finch brains provide an experimental system that should allow correlation of biological aspects of a neurotrophic agent with measurable behavioural traits. Our results show that the roles of IGFs in the adult brain are not limited to mammals. We presented a transgenic mouse model with liver-specific overexpression of IGFBP-1, which shows growth deficiency and abnormal CNS development. Comparison with the phenotypes of IGF transgenic mice, including those with brain-specific expression, showed that peripheral IGFBP overexpression can produce similar CNS defects. Further exploration of our transgenic model may provide new insights into the relationship between endocrine and paracrine effects of the IGFs on CNS development.

Acknowledgements

This work was supported by INSERM, The European Communities Science Programme (M.H.), PHS grants MH 18343 and 53542, and NSF grant IBN-9319638. Experiments on songbirds have been carried out in the laboratory of

F. Nottebohm, Rockefeller University New York, in collaboration with C. Scharff and E. D. Jarvis. We would like to thank C. Duyckaerts (Laboratoire de Neuropathologie, Hôpital de la Salpêtrière, Paris) for histopathological expertise of the brains of IGFBP-1 Tg mice, C. Scharff and E. D. Jarvis for critically reading the manuscript, and D. Seurin (INSERM U.142), C. Chong and M. Grossman (Rockefeller University) for expert technical assistance.

References

1. Efstratiadis A (1994) IGFs and dwarf mice: Genetic and epigenetic control of embryonic growth. In: Sizonenko PC, Aubert ML, Vassalli J-D (eds) Frontiers in Endocrinology: Developmental Endocrinology, Vol 6. Ares-Serono Symposia, Rome, pp 27-42
2. Bartlett WP, Li X-S, Williams M, Benkovic S (1991) Localization of insulin-like growth factor-1 mRNA in murine central nervous system during postnatal development. Dev Biol 147:239-250
3. Marks JL, Porte Jr D, Baskin DG (1991) Localization of type I insulin-like growth factor receptor messenger RNA in the adult rat brain by in situ hybridization. Mol Endocrinol 5:1158-1168
4. Bondy CA, Werner H, Roberts Jr CT, LeRoith D (1992) Cellular pattern of type-I insulin-like growth factor receptor gene expression during maturation of the rat brain: comparison with insulin-like growth factors I and II. Neuroscience 46:909-923
5. Couce ME, Weatherington AJ, McGinty J (1992) Expression of insulin-like growth factor-II (IGF-II) and IGF-II mannose-6-phosphate receptor in the rat hippocampus: an in situ hybridization and immunocytochemical study. Endocrinology 131:1636-1642
6. Logan A, Gonzalez A-M, Hill DJ, Berry M, Gregson NA, Baird A (1994) Coordinated pattern of expression and localization of insulin-like growth factor-II (IGF-II) and IGF-binding protein-2 in the adult rat brain. Endocrinology 135:2255-2264
7. Baker J, Liu J-P, Robertson EJ, Efstratiadis A (1993) Role of insulin-like growth factors in embryonic and postnatal growth. Cell 75:73-82
8. Liu J-P, Baker J, Perkins AS, Robertson EJ, Efstratiadis A (1993) Mice carrying null mutations of the genes encoding insulin-like growth factor I (Igf-1) and type 1 IGF receptor (Igf1r). Cell 75:59-72
9. Powell-Braxton L, Hollingshead P, Warburton C, Dowd M, Pitts-Meek S, Dalton D, Gillett STA (1993) IGF-I is required for normal embryonic growth in mice. Genes Dev 7:2609-2617
10. Beck KD, Powell-Braxton L, Widmer H-R, Valverde J, Hefti F (1995) Igf1 gene disruption results in reduced brain size, CNS hypomyelination, and loss of hippocampal granule and striatal parvalbumin-containing neurons. Neuron 14:717-730
11. De Chiara TM, Efstratiadis A, Robertson EJ (1990) A growth-deficiency phenotype in heterozygous mice carrying an insulin-like growth factor II gene disrupted by targeting. Nature 345:78-80
12. Ye P, Carson J, D'Ercole AJ (1995) In vivo actions of insulin-like growth factor-I (IGF-I) on brain myelination: studies of IGF-I and IGF binding protein-1 (IGFBP-1) transgenic mice. J Neurosci 15:7344-7356
13. D'Ercole AJ, Ye P, Dai Z (1995) Human insulin-like growth factor binding protein-1 (hIGFBP-1) transgenic mice: insights into hIGFBP-1 regulation and actions. Prog Growth Factor Res 6:417-423
14. D'Mello SR, Galli C, Ciotti T, Calissano P (1993) Induction of apoptosis in cerebellar

granule neurons by low potassium: inhibition of death by insulin-like growth factor I and cAMP. Proc Natl Acad Sci USA 90:10989-10993

15. D'Mello SR, Borodezt K, Soltoff SP (1997) Insulin-like growth factor and potassium depolarization maintain neuronal survival by distinct pathways: possible involvement of PI 3-kinase in IGF-1 signaling. J Neurosci 17:1548-1560

16. Galli C, Meucci O, Scorziello A, Werge TM, Calissano P, Schettini G (1995) Apoptosis in cerebellar granule cells is blocked by high KCl, forskolin, and IGF-I through distinct mechanisms of action: the involvement of intracellular calcium and RNA synthesis. J Neurosci 15:1172-1179

17. Aguado F, Sánchez-Franco F, Caciedo L, Fernández T, Rodrigo J, Martinez-Murillo R (1992) Subcellular localization of insulin-like growth factor I (IGF-I) in Purkinje cells of the adult rat: an immunocytochemical study. Neurosci Lett 135:171-174

18. Aguado F, Sánchez-Franco F, Rodrigo J, Caciedo L, Martinez-Murillo R (1994) Insulin-like growth factor-I immunoreactive peptide in adult human cerebellar Purkinje cells: co-localization with low-affinity nerve growth factor receptor. Neurosci Lett 135:171-174

19. Guan J, Williams C, Gunning M, Mallard C, Gluckman P (1993) The effects of IGF-1 treatment after hypoxic-ischemic brain injury in adult rats. J Cereb Blood Flow Metab 13:609-616

20. Guan J, Williams CE, Skinner SJM, Mallard EC, Gluckman PD (1996) The effects of insulin-like growth factor (IGF)-1, IGF-2, and des-IGF-1 on neuronal loss after hypoxic-ischemic brain injury in adult rats: evidence for a role for IGF binding proteins. Endocrinology 137:893-898

21. Beilharz EJ, Bassett NS, Sirimanne, ES, Williams CE, Gluckman PD (1994) Insulin-like growth factor II is induced during wound repair following hypoxic-ischemic injury in the developing rat brain. Mol Brain Res 29:81-91

22. Beilharz EJ, Williams CE, Dragunow M, Sirimanne ES, Gluckman PD (1995) Mechanisms of delayed cell death following hypoxic-ischemic injury in the immature rat: evidence for apoptosis during selective neuronal loss. Mol Brain Res 29:1-14

23. Johnston BM, Mallard EC, Williams CE, Gluckman PD (1996) Insulin-like growth factor-1 is a potent neuronal rescue agent after hypoxic-ischemic injury in fetal lambs. J Clin Invest 97:300-308

24. Singleton JR, Dixit VM, Feldman E (1996) Type I insulin-like growth factor receptor activation regulates apoptotic proteins. J Biol Chem 271:31791-31794

25. Guthrie KM, Nguyen T, Gall CM (1995) Insulin-like growth factor-1 mRNA is increased in deafferented hippocampus: spatiotemporal correspondance of a trophic event with axon sprouting. J Comp Neurol 352:147-160

26. Quiroga S, Garofalo RS, Pfenninger KHAD (1995) Insulin-like growth factor I receptors of fetal brain are enriched in nerve growth cones and contain a beta-subunit variant. Proc Natl Acad Sci USA 92:4309-4312

27. Mascotti FD, Càceres A, Pfenniger KH, Quiroga S (1997) Expression and distribution of IGF-1 receptors containing a β-subunit (βgc) in developing neurons. J Neurosci 17:1447-1459

28. Doré S, Kar S, Quirion R (1997) Emploi thérapeutique de l'IGF-I dans le traitement des maladies neurodégénératives. Méd Sciences 13:557-565

29. Carson MJ, Behringer RR, Brinster RL, McMorris FA (1993) Insulin-like growth factor I increases brain growth and central nervous system myelination in transgenic mice. Neuron 10:729-740

30. D'Ercole AJ, Dai Z, Xing Y, Boney C, Wilkie MB, Lauder JM, Han VKM, Clemmons DR (1994) Brain growth retardation due to the expression of human insulin like growth

factor binding protein-1 in transgenic mice: an in vivo model for the analysis of IGF function in the brain. Dev Brain Res 82:213-222

31. Gutierrez-Ospina G, Calikoglu AS, Ye P, D'Ercole AJ (1996) *In vivo* effects of insulin-like growth factor-I on the development of sensory pathways: analysis of the primary somatic sensory cortex (S1) of transgenic mice. Endocrinology 137:5484-5492

32. Rajkumar K, Barron D, Lewitt MS, Murphy LJ (1995) Growth retardation and hyperglycemia in insulin-like growth factor binding protein-1 transgenic mice. Endocrinology 136:4029-4034

33. Giacobini MMJ, Zetterström RH, Young D, Hoffer B, Sara V, Olson L (1995) IGF-1 influences olfactory bulb maturation. Evidence from anti-IGF-1 antibody treatment of developing grafts in oculo. Dev Brain Res 84:67-76

34. Lois C, Alvarez-Buylla A (1994) Long-distance neuronal migration in the adult mammalian brain. Science 264:1145-1148

35. Lois C, Garcia-Verdugo J-M, Alvarez-Buylla A (1996) Chain migration of neuronal precursors. Science 271:978-981

36. Castro-Alamancos MA, Torres-Aleman I (1994) Learning of the conditioned eyeblink response is impaired by an antisense insulin-like growth factor I oligonucleotide. Proc Natl Acad Sci USA 91:10203-10207

37. Woods KA, Camacho-Hübner C, Savage MO, Clark AJL (1995) Intrauterine growth retardation and postnatal growth failure associated with deletion of the insulin-like growth factor-I gene. New Engl J Med 335:1363-1365

38. Ayer-Le Lièvre C, Stahlbom P-A, Sara V (1991) Expression of IGF-I and -II mRNA in the brain and facial region of the rat fetus. Development 111:105-115

39. Bondy C, Lee W-H (1993) Correlation between insulin-like growth factor (IGF)-binding protein 5 and IGF-I gene expression during brain development. J Neurosci 13:5092-5104

40. Holzenberger M, Lapointe F, Leibovici M, Ayer-Le Lièvre C (1996) The avian IGF type 1 receptor: cDNA analysis and *in situ* hybridization reveal conserved sequence elements and expression patterns relevant for the development of the nervous system. Dev Brain Res 97:76-87

41. Graziadei PPC, Monti-Graziadei GA (1985) Neurogenesis and plasticity of the olfactory sensory neurons. Ann N Y Acad Sci 457:127-142

42. D'Ercole AJ, Ye P, Gutierrez-Ospina G (1996) Use of transgenic mice for understanding the physiology of insulin-like growth factors. Horm Res 45 (Suppl):5-7

43. Barde Y-A (1989) Trophic factors and neuronal survival. Neuron 2:1525-1534

44. Nottebohm F, Kelley DB, Paton JA (1982) Connections of vocal control nuclei in the canary telencephalon. J Comp Neurol 207:344-357

45. Nottebohm F, O'Loughlin B, Gould K, Yohay K, Alvarez-Buylla A (1994) The life span of new neurons in a song control nucleus of the adult canary brain depends on time of year when these cells are born. Proc Natl Acad Sci USA 91:7849-7853

46. Alvarez-Buylla A (1992) Neurogenesis and plasticity in the CNS of adult birds. Exp Neurol 115:110-114

47. Holzenberger M, Erich DJ, Chong C, Grossman M, Nottebohm F, Scharff C (1997) Selective expression of insulin-like growth factor II in the songbird brain. J Neurosci 17:6974-6987

48. Kirn JR, Alvarez-Buylla A, Nottebohm F (1991) Production and survival of projection neurons in a forebrain vocal center of adult male canaries. J Neurosci 11:1756-1762

49. Kirn J, O'Loughlin B, Kasparian S, Nottebohm F (1994) Cell death and neuronal recruitment in the high vocal center of adult male canaries are temporally related to changes in song. Proc Natl Acad Sci USA 91:7844-7848

50. Nordeen KW, Nordeen EJ (1988) Projection neurons within a vocal motor pathway are born during song learning in zebra finches. Nature 334:149-151

51. Alvarez-Buylla A, Kirn JR, Nottebohm F (1990) Birth of projection neurons in adult avian brain may be related to perceptual or motor learning. Science 249:1444-1446

52. Qin-Wei Y, Johnson J, Prevette D, Oppenheim RW (1994) Cell death of spinal motoneurons in the chick embryo following deafferentiation: rescue effects of tissue extracts, soluble proteins, and neurotrophic agents. J Neurosci 14:7629-7640

53. Barnea A, Nottebohm F (1994) Seasonal recruitment of hippocampal neurons in adult free-ranging black-capped chickadees. Proc Natl Acad Sci USA 91:11217-11221

54. Barnea A, Nottebohm F (1996) Recruitment and replacement of hippocampal neurons in young and adult chickadees: an addition to the theory of hippocampal learning. Proc Natl Acad Sci USA 93:714-718

55. Reinhardt RR, Bondy CA (1994) Insulin-like growth factors cross the blood-brain barrier. Endocrinology 135:1753-1761

56. Roghani M, Lassarre C, Zapf J, Povoa G, Binoux M (1991) Two insulin-like growth factor binding proteins are responsible for the selective affinity for IGF-II of cerebrospinal fluid binding proteins. J Clin Endocrinol Metab 73:658-666

57. Roghani M, Segovia B, Whitechurch O, Binoux M (1991) Purification from cerebrospinal fluid of insulin-like growth factor binding proteins (IGFBPs). Isolation of IGFBP-2, an altered form of IGFBP-3 and a new IGFBP species. Growth Regul 1:125-130

58. Stylianopoulou F, Efstratiadis A, Herbert J, Pintar J (1988) Pattern of the insulin-like growth factor II gene expression during rat embryogenesis. Development 103:497-506

59. Sullivan KA, Feldman EL (1994) Immunohistochemical localization of insulin-like growth factor-II (IGF-II) and IGF-binding protein-2 during development in the rat brain. Endocrinology 135:540-547

60. Gay E, Seurin D, Babajko S, Doublier S, Cazillis M, Binoux M (1997) Liver-specific expression of human insulin-like growth factor binding protein-1 (IGFBP-1) in transgenic mice: repercussions on reproduction, ante- and perinatal mortality and postnatal growth. Endocrinology 138:2937-2947

61. D'Ercole AJ, Ye P, Caligoklu AS, Gutierrez-Ospina G (1996) The role of the insulin-like growth factors in the central nervous system. Mol Neurobiol 13:227-255

62. Kühn R, Schwenk F, Aguet M, Rajewsky K (1995) Inducible gene targeting in mice. Science 269:1427-1429

63. Tsien JZ, Chen DF, Gerber D, Tom C, Mercer, EH, Anderson DJ, Mayford M, Kandel ER, Tonegawa S (1996) Subregion- and cell type-restricted gene knockout in mousebrain. Cell 87:1317-1326

64. Rajewsky K, Gu H, Kühn R, Betz UAK, Müller W, Roes J, Schwenk F (1996) Conditional gene targeting. J Clin Invest 98:600-603

65. Gossen M, Freundlieb S, Bender G, Müller G, Hillen W, Bujard H (1995) Transcriptional activation by tetracyclins in mammalian cells. Science 268:1766-1769

66. Kistner A, Gossen M, Zimmermann F, Jerecic J, Ullmer C, Lübbert H, Bujard H (1996) Doxycycline-mediated quantitative and tissue-specific control of gene expression in transgenic mice. Proc Natl Acad Sci USA 93:10933-10938

The Insulin-like Growth Factor-I Receptor and the Central Nervous System: Mechanisms Involved in the Prevention of Apoptosis

D. Le Roith, M. Párrizas, V. A. Blakesley

Introduction

Apoptosis or programmed cell death is an essential element in the regulation and behavior of mammalian cells [1, 2]. The process is a genetically controlled response for cells to commit suicide and is orchestrated by mechanisms involving various proteins. The purpose of apoptosis is to kill unwanted cells. This process is important in the developing nervous system where a large excess of redundant neurons die off during the period when synapses are being formed between the neurons and their target cells [3, 4]. Apparently, the surviving neurons represent those that receive survival signals from the target cells. Apoptosis is also important in the nervous system following injury. Traumatic injury to the nervous system initially causes necrosis at the injury site, followed by secondary processes which cause spreading of the damage beyond this initial site of damage [5]. This secondary event is apoptosis, and occurs hours after the initial injury. Following spinal cord injury, for example, the apoptotic cells were found to be oligodendrocytes in the spinal white matter as well as in the fiber tracts, which became demyelinated as a result of apoptosis. The process of apoptosis in this model apparently occurs secondary to the release of cytokines such as tumor necrosis factor and certain interleukins. In a separate study of hypoxic-ischemic injury to the brain in rats, insulin-like growth factor-I (IGF-I) was protective against neuronal cell death [6].

A second, important role for apoptosis is as a defense mechanism [7]. Invasion by viruses may trigger cell suicide to prevent spread of the virus to neighboring cells. Apoptosis is also critical for the normal functioning of the immune system, where certain cells need to be removed lest they attack normal cells. Additionally, by preventing the onset or progression of tumors, apoptosis is the antithesis of cellular proliferation and can impair cellular proliferation [8]. Finally, apoptosis is a distinctive feature of the aging process, in which it leads to loss of essential cells and impairment of normal functioning of specialized organs.

Apoptosis is a highly ordered process that may be characterized by nuclear

Diabetes Branch, NIDDK, National Institutes of Health, Bethesda, MD 20892-1770 USA

changes including chromatin condensation, fragmentation and margination as well as internucleosomal DNA cleavage which gives rise to the characteristic DNA laddering [9]. In addition, there is cytoskeletal disruption, shrinkage of the cell and membrane blebbing, resulting in membrane-bound apoptotic bodies. The process often results in an undesirable inflammatory response [10].

At present there are a number of known signaling pathways which are involved in apoptotic processes. The complexity of these systems is rapidly becoming very evident as new proteins and signaling complexes are shown to impact on the activation or prevention of apoptosis. Apparently, individual tissues and organ systems use different combinations of these signaling pathways to achieve the final result of apoptosis. Presumably such complexity allows for specialized control of cellular death versus cellular survival, proliferation and differentiation.

Insulin-like growth factors (IGF-I and IGF-II), like several other growth factors, prevent apoptosis in a number of different cells and tissues [11-13]. The mechanisms involved in these effects are not well defined and rightly form the basis of current research projects being carried out by a number of different investigators. In this review we describe the current knowledge of the signaling pathways whereby IGF-I inhibits apoptosis.

The MAP Kinase and PI 3'-Kinase Pathways

The IGFs exert their biological effects by binding and activating the IGF-I receptor, which is ubiquitiously expressed. The IGF-I receptor is a hetero-tetrameric protein with marked aminoacid and structural similarity to the insulin receptor [14, 15]. The IGFs bind to the extracellular α subunits and trigger the tyrosine kinase activity which is found in the cytoplasmic region of the β subunit. The initial response to the binding of the ligand is autophosphorylation of the receptor followed by tyrosine phosphorylation of two major substrates of the receptor, namely insulin receptor substrate (IRS) 1 and 2. Tyrosylphosphorylated IRS-1 and IRS-2 then interact with a number of *src* homology 2 (SH2) domain-containing proteins (Fig. 1). These include p85, the regulatory subunit of phosphoinositide (PI) 3'-kinase, the tyrosine phosphatase PTP1D (or Syp), the gaunine-nucleotide exhange protein GRB2, the Ras-binding protein GAP, and the proto-oncogene products Crk and Nck [15, 16]. SHC is also phosphorylated directly by the IGF-I receptor and binds the GRB2/Sos complex. These interactions lead to activation of downstream signaling proteins and kinases, all arranged in signaling cascades. For the IGF-I-mediated response, the significant cascades are the Ras/Raf/mitogen-activated protein (MAP) kinase pathway and the PI 3'-kinase pathway [15].

To determine the possible role of these signaling pathways in the action of IGF-I on the inhibition of apoptosis, we utilized the well-characterized model of differentiated pheochromocytoma PC12 cells. These cells differentiate in the presence of serum and nerve growth factor (NGF), and then undergo apoptosis

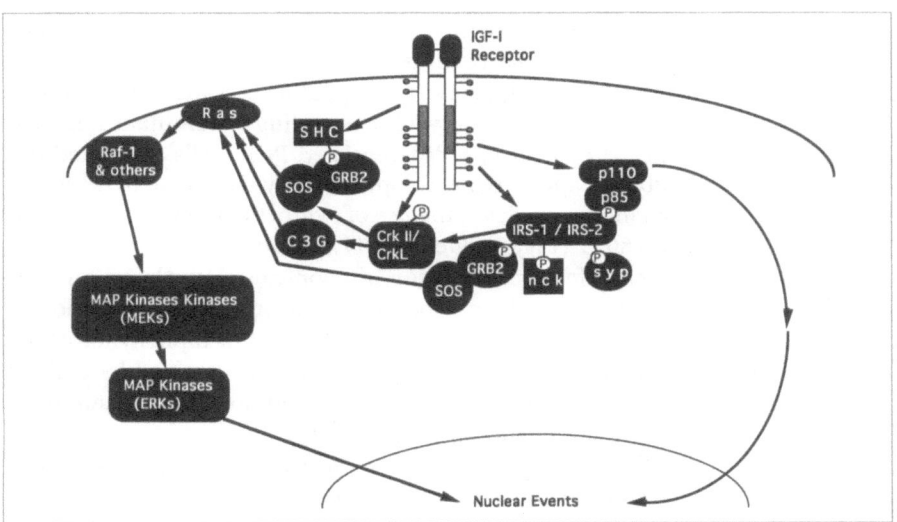

Fig. 1. Major signaling pathways mediating the effects of the activated insulin-like growth factor-I receptor

following the removal of serum and NGF [17]. Apoptosis, clearly seen as DNA laddering (Fig. 2, lanes 2, 4, 6 and 8), is inhibited by the addition of physiological concentrations of IGF-I (10 nM) (Fig. 2, lanes 1, 3, 5 and 7).

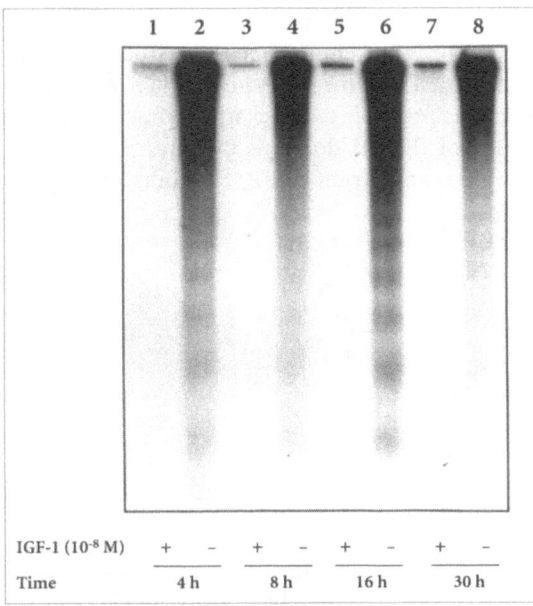

Fig. 2. Apoptosis developing in PC12 cells following serum and growth factor withdrawal for 4-30 hours. Apoptosis is seen as laddering of the DNA and is inhibited by the addition of IGF-I alone in the cell culture medium at time 0

The Ras/Raf/MAP kinase pathway may be inhibited by multiple interventions. Expression of dominant negative proteins will inhibit activation of downstream enzymes, thereby disrupting the normal signaling cascades. For example, transient transfection of an expression vector encoding a dominant negative MAPK/ERK kinase (MEK) protein into differentiated PC12 cells abrogated the effect of IGF-I on inhibiting apoptosis. A complementary technique by which to disrupt the crucial signaling cascades is the use of synthetic inhibitors of several of these kinases. PD098059 (Fig. 3) specifically inhibits MEK and similarly inhibits IGF-I's biological effect on inhibition of apoptosis (Fig. 4) [18-20]. Cell survival has also been determined by manual cell counting and the estimation of cell number using an MTT (3-(4,5-dimethylthiazol-2-yl)-2,5-diphenyltetrazolium bromide) assay. Decreased survival of PC12 cells, as determined by both of these methods, closely paralleled the responses to apoptosis as measured by DNA laddering and in situ staining for apoptotic nuclei.

The role of the PI 3'-kinase pathway was also investigated using a dominant negative p85 molecule stably expressed in PC12 cells [21]. The blockade of PI 3'-kinase diminished the IGF-I protective effect from apoptosis. The fungal metabolite wortmannin and the synthetic compound LY294002, the first a general inhibitor and the second a specific inhibitor of the p110 catalytic subunit of PI 3'-kinase, inhibited IGF-I protection from apoptosis (Fig. 4) [22].

Thus, in differentiated PC12 cells both the Ras/Raf/MAP kinase and the PI 3'-kinase pathways are apparently involved in mediating anti-apoptotic IGF-I action. Since these pathways also interact with other signaling cascades, the results of studies cited do not exclude the role of other similar signaling pathways such as the p38 and JNK stress-related pathways [23]. Indeed, Heidenreich and Kummer [24] have demonstrated that apoptosis in cultured fetal neurons is associated with increased p38 MAP kinase activity. Another critical protein in the apoptotic pathway is the recently identified proto-oncogene product Akt (also called protein kinase B-α or RAC-α), which contains a pleckstrin homology (PH) domain. Based on the known property of the PH domains of other proteins to bind lipids, Akt is a potential downstream target for PI 3'-kinase (Fig. 5).

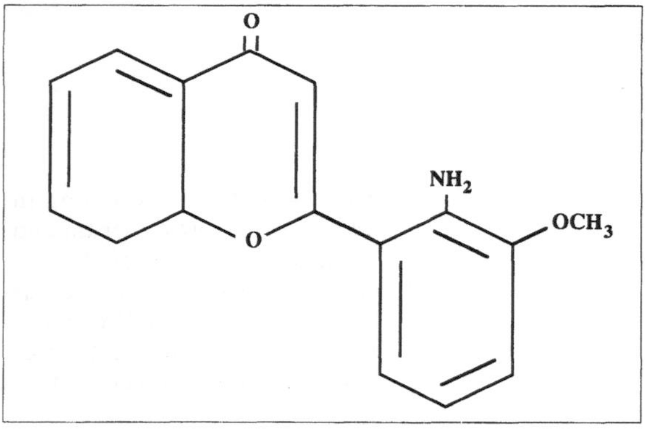

Fig. 3. Structure of the specific MEK inhibitor PD098059

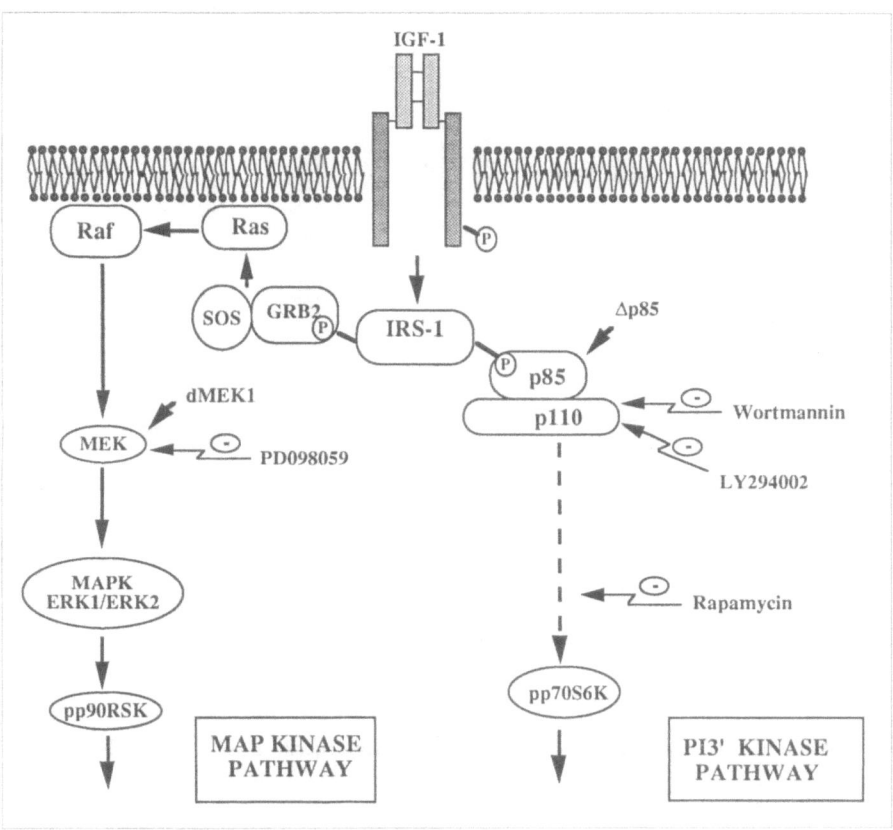

Fig. 4. Signaling pathways inhibited in PC12 cells. Wortmannin and LY294002 are inhibitors of the catalytic subunit of PI 3'-kinase (p110) whereas Δ p85 is a dominant-negative inhibitor that interferes with the normal interaction of p85 with tyrosine phosphorylated IRS-1. MEK is inhibited by PD098059, a synthetic inhibitor, and by the expression of a dominant-negative MEK protein (dMEK1)

Activation of Akt occurs in response to increased lipid kinase activity of PI 3'-kinase following stimulation by growth factors. Furthermore, the PI 3'-kinase inhibitors wortmannin and LY294002 block growth factor activation of Akt [25, 26]. Specifically, IGF-I enhances Akt activity 20-50 fold with concommitant phosphorylation of residues Thr-308 and Ser-473 of Akt. Primary cultures of cerebellar neurons undergo apoptosis in the absence of survival factors. Addition of physiologic concentrations of IGF-I inhibits this apoptosis. The Ras/Raf/MAP kinase pathway is not involved in mediating this protective effect. However, IGF-I stimulates activation of PI 3'-kinase, Akt and p70S6 kinase, and each of these activities is inhibited by wortmannin. However, p70S6 kinase is apparently not important in mediating the effect of IGF-I since rapamycin fails to inhibit the IGF-I effect on preventing apoptosis.

Besides delineating some of the specific IGF-I-stimulated functions of sever-

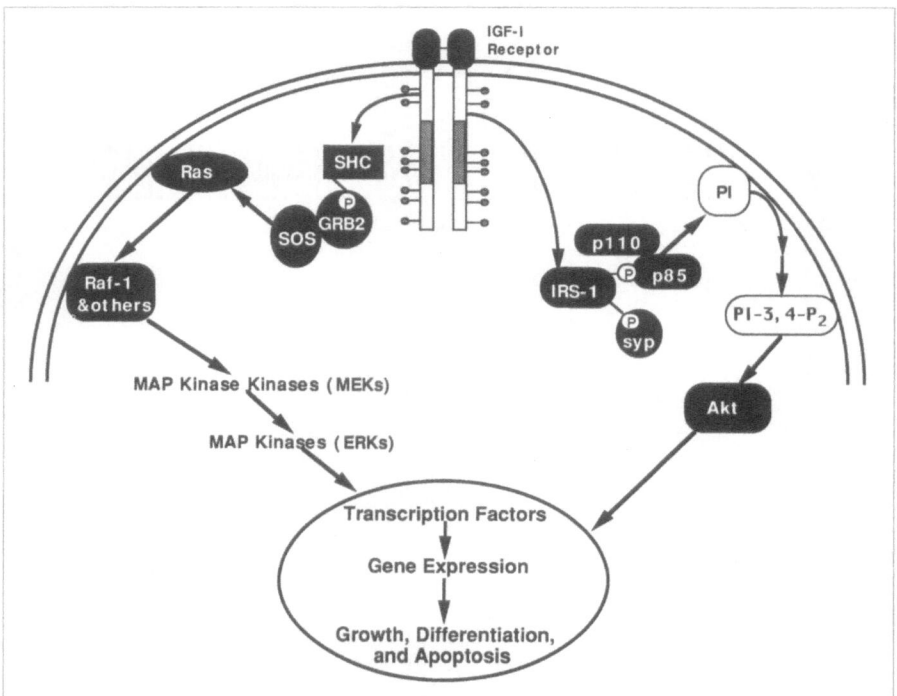

Fig. 5. Signaling pathways including Akt/PKB, a recently described substrate of the insulin and IGF-I receptor signaling cascades

al proteins and signaling cascades resulting in protection from apoptosis, the results cited above suggest cell-type specific utilization of the known anti-apop-totic pathways.

The Bcl-2 Family of Survival/Death Proteins

The first member of the Bcl-2 family of proteins was identified in *Caenorhabditis elegans* as the *ced-9* gene product which mediates developmentally related cell death. Presently, the mammalian ced-9-related proteins include Bcl-2, Bcl-X, Bax, Bad and Bak, and new members are rapidly being discovered [27]. Two of the known mammalian proteins, Bcl-2 and Bcl-X$_L$ (the long form), negatively regulate apoptosis; instead Bcl-X$_S$ (the short form), Bax and Bad induce apoptosis. While the exact mechanism of action is not well understood, it has been shown that het-erodimers of Bcl-2 or Bcl-X$_L$ with Bax or Bad inhibit the activity of Bax or Bad to induce apoptosis (Fig. 6).

To determine whether the IGFs may inhibit apoptosis via this family of pro-teins, we studied human 293 embryonic kidney cells which undergo apoptosis in serum-free medium. IGF-I induced the expression of Bcl-X$_L$ in a time- and

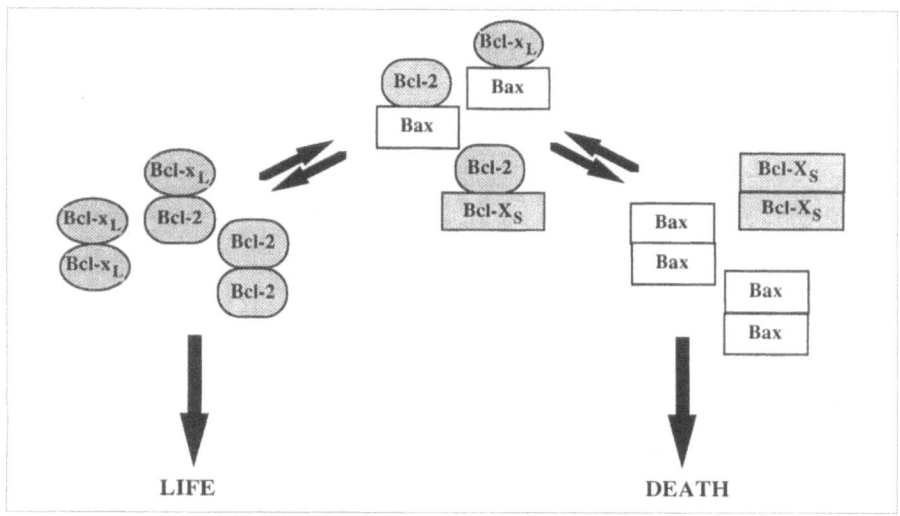

Fig. 6. The Bcl-2 family of proteins. Bcl-2 inhibits apoptosis, as does the long form of the Bcl-X (Bcl-X$_L$). In contrast, the short form (Bcl-X$_S$) enhances apoptosis, as do Bax and Bad

dose-dependent manner (Fig. 7a,b). An increase of Bcl-X$_L$ mRNA preceded an increase in protein levels [28]. In SH-SY5Y neuroblastoma cells, mannitol-induced hyperosmotic stress was associated with alterations in the levels of the Bcl-2 and Bcl-X$_L$ proteins [29]. The reduction in the levels of these anti-apoptotic proteins was overcome by treatment with IGF-II or overexpression of the IGF-I receptor. These results support the hypothesis that long-term effects of the IGFs on preventing apoptosis may be mediated via these proteins.

Thus, in both 293 and SH-SY5Y cells the proteins of the Bcl-2 family are involved in the inhibition of apoptosis mediated by activation of the IGF-I receptor and its down-stream signaling pathways. These results support the hypothesis tendered above that in each cell type specific pathways are involved in modulating apoptosis and that these pathways may also be specific for the particular growth factor mediating the effect.

Other proteins may transduce the effects of the IGFs including the interleukin-1β-converting enzyme (ICE)-related proteases, of which there are several described members [30]. Yama/CPP32 and ICE/LAP3 are cleaved and activated upon hyperosmotic stress in SH-SY5Y cells. This cleavage is prevented by IGF-II treatment. Activation of these serine proteases is dependent on cleavage of the precursor ICE proteases. Cleaved ICE proteases subsequently cleave the 116 kDa nuclear protein poly (ADP-ribose) polymerase (PARP) yielding an 85 kDa apoptotic protein fragment. Thus, PARP protein fragments are yet another marker of apoptosis. The exact IGF-I receptor-activated pathways that integrate at the level of the ICE proteases have yet to be fully described; however, studies to date indicate that the anti-apoptotic mechanisms of the IGFs are multifaceted. It is likely that regulation of the signaling via the ICE proteases is also complex and tightly controlled.

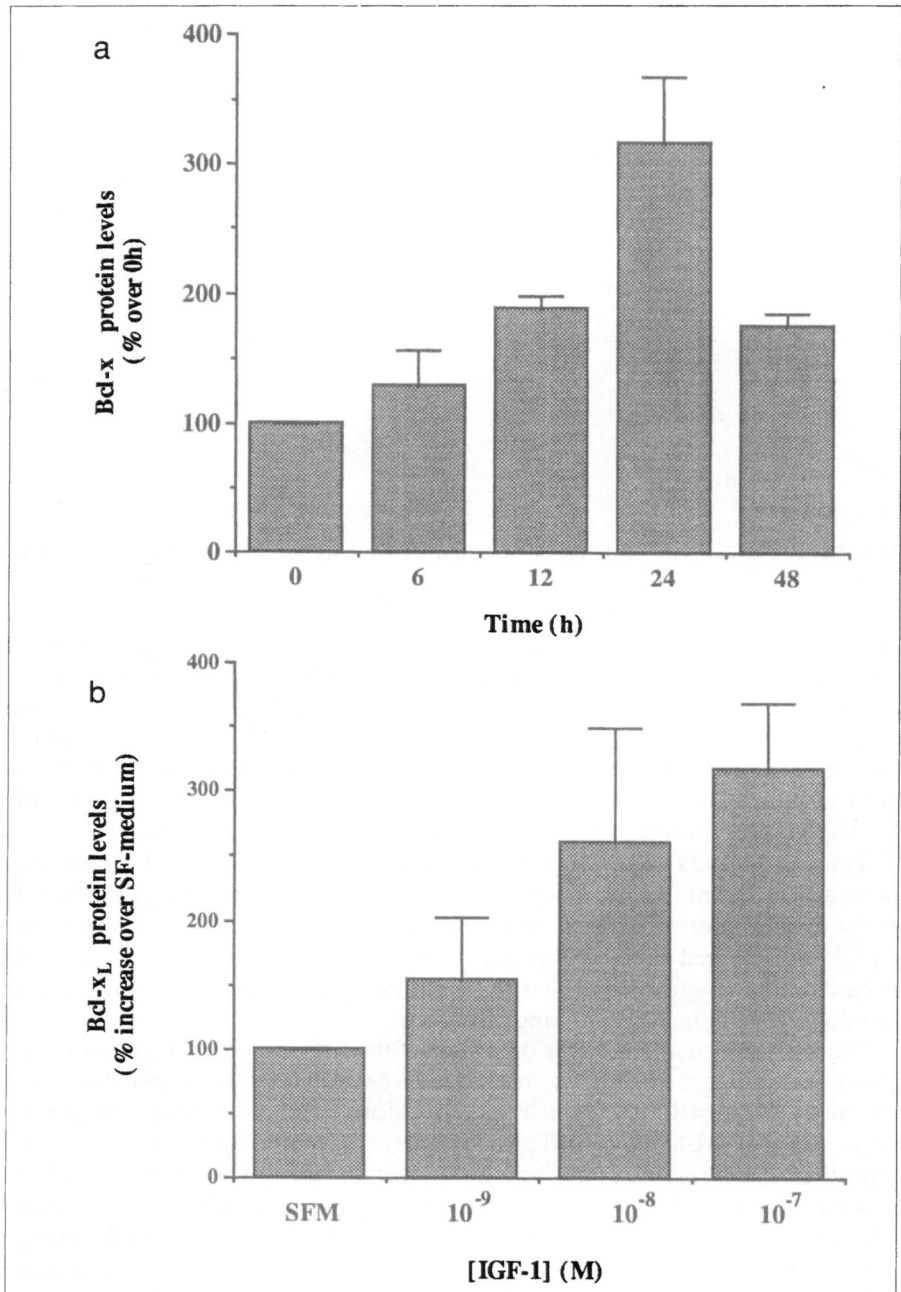

Fig. 7. a Time-dependent, increased expression of Bcl-X$_L$ protein induced by IGF-I. **b** Dose-dependent, increased expression of Bcl-X$_L$ protein induced by IGF-I. *SF*, serum-free; *SFM*, serum-free medium

Expression of the IGF-I Receptor and Apoptosis

The levels of expression of the IGF-I receptor are important in determining cell survival or cell death [31-33]. Antisense strategies and dominant negative mutant receptors reduce the expression or function of the normal IGF-I receptor and result in increased apoptosis in cancer cells and tumors. Overexpression of IGF-I receptors, on the other hand, protects against apoptosis.

Expression of the IGF-I receptor is regulated by numerous growth factors and tumor suppressor gene products. Basic fibroblast growth factor and platelet-derived growth factor increase expression of the receptor at the level of transcription, whereas WT-1 and p53 inhibit the expression by direct interaction with the promoter of the IGF-I receptor. In the case of p53, the reduction in IGF-I receptors enhanced the sensitivity of these cells to apoptosis [34-36].

Conclusions and Future Directions

This review has described results of recently published reports on the signaling pathways involved in IGF-I inhibition of apoptosis. As this is an exciting and topical subject with importance to the understanding of a number of physiological and pathological states, one can anticipate reports of more studies in the near future. In addition it is predicted that there will be many more pathways described that mediate apoptosis. It seems obvious that a complete understanding of the mechanisms involved in the IGFs' anti-apoptotic effect will help elucidate the complex interactions occurring within the cell and potentially will guide the design of therapeutic agents with high benefit-to-risk ratios. However, the eminently more important biological question to be answered is exactly which factors control the balance between apoptosis and cell cycling resulting in cellular proliferation. An extension of the elucidation of the interactions between these factors would also help answer this basic biological question. The perturbation of this programmed balance of cellular proliferation and cell death is critical in the processes of development and aging and in diseases such as cancer and numerous neurological and neuromuscular degenerative disorders.

References

1. Kerr JFR, Wylie AH, Currie AR (1972) Apoptosis: a basic biological phenomenon with wide ranging implications in tissue kinetics. Br J Cancer 26:239-257
2. Wylie AH, Kerr JFR, Currie AR (1986) Cell death: the significance of apoptosis. Int Rev Cytol 68:251-306
3. Raff MC, Barres BA, Burne JF, Coles HS, Ishizaki Y, Jacobson MI (1993) Programmed cell death and the control of cell survival: lessons from the nervous system. Science 262:695-700
4. Oppenheim RW (1991) Cell death during development of the nervous system. Annu Rev Neurosci 14:453-450

5. Crowe MJ, Bresnahan JC, Shuman SL, Masters JN, Beattie MS (1997) Apoptosis and delayed degeneration after spinal cord injury in rats and monkeys. Nat Med 3:73-77

6. Gluckman P, Klempt N, Guan J et al (1992) A role for IGF-1 in the rescue of CNS neurons following hypoxic-ischemic injury. Biochem Biophys Res Comm 182:593-599

7. Thompson CB (1995) Apoptosis in the pathogenesis and treatment of disease. Science 267:1456-1462

8. Resnicoff M, Abraham D, Yutanawiboonchai W et al (1995) The insulin-like growth factor I receptor protects tumor cells from apoptosis in vivo. Cancer Res 55:2463-2469

9. Bursch W, Kleine L, Tenniswood M (1990) The biochemistry of cell death by apoptosis. Biochem Cell Biol 68:1071-1074

10. Pittman RN, Wang S, DiBenedetto A, Mills JC (1993) A system for characterizing cellular and molecular events in programmed neuronal cell death. J Neurosci 13:3669-3680

11. D'Mello SR, Galli C, Ciotti T, Calissano P (1993) Induction of apoptosis in cerebellar granule neurons by low potassium: Inhibition of death by insulin-like growth factor I and cAMP. Proc Natl Acad Sci USA 90:10989-10993

12. Galli C, Meucci O, Scorziello A, Werge TM, Calissano P, Schettini G (1995) Apoptosis in cerebellar granule cells is blocked by high KCl, forskolin and IGF-1 through distinct mechanisms of action: the involvement of intracellular calcium and RNA synthesis. J Neurosci 15:1172-1179

13. Harrington EA, Bennett MR, Fanidi A, Evan GI (1994) c-Myc-induced apoptosis in fibroblasts is inhibited by specific cytokines. EMBO J 13:3286-3295

14. Ullrich A, Gray A, Tam AW et al (1986) Insulin-like growth factor-1 receptor primary structure: comparison with insulin receptor suggests structural determinants that define functional specificity. EMBO J 5:2503-2512

15. LeRoith D, Werner H, Beitner-Johnson D, Roberts CT Jr (1995) Molecular and cellular aspects of the insulin-like growth factor-I receptor. Endocr Rev 16:143-163

16. Backer JM, Myers MG Jr, Shoelson SE et al (1992) Phosphatidylinositol 3' kinase is activated by association with IRS-1 during insulin stimulation. EMBO J 11:3469-3479

17. Yao R, Cooper GM (1995) Requirement for phosphatidylinositol-3' kinase in the prevention of apoptosis by nerve growth factor. Science 267:2003-2200

18. Allesi DR, Cunda A, Cohen P, Dudley DT, Saltiel A (1995) PD098059 is a specific inhibitor of the activation of mitogen-activated protein kinase kinase *in vitro* and *in vivo*. J Biol Chem 270:27489-27495

19. Dudley DT, Pang L, Decker SJ, Bridges AJ, Saltiel AR (1995) A synthetic inhibitor of the mitogen-activated protein kinase cascade. Proc Natl Acad Sci USA 92:7686-7689

20. Párrizas M, Saltiel AR, Le Roith D (1997) Insulin-like growth factor-I inhibits apoptosis using the phosphatidylinositol 3'-kinase and mitogen-activated protein kinase pathways. J Biol Chem 272:154-161

21. Dhand R, Hara K, Hiles I et al (1994) PI 3'-kinase: structural and functional analysis of intersubunit interactions. EMBO J 13:511-521

22. Vlahos CJ, Matter WF, Hui KY, Brown RF (1994) A specific inhibitor of phosphatidylinositol 3'-kinase, 2-(4-morpholinyl-)-8-phenyl-4H-1-benzopyran-4-one (LY294002). J Biol Chem 269:5241-5248

23. Xia Z, Dickens M, Raingeaud J, Davis RJ, Greenberg ME (1995) Opposing effects of ERK and JNK-p38 MAP kinases on apoptosis. Science 270:1326-1331

24. Heidenreich KA, Kummer JL (1996) Inhibition of p38 mitogen-activated protein kinase by insulin in cultured fetal neurons. J Biol Chem 271:9891-9894

25. Kulik G, Klippel A, Weber MJ (1997) Antiapoptotic signalling by the insulin-like

growth factor I receptor, phosphatidylinositol 3'-kinase and Akt. Mol Cell Biol 17:1595-1606

26. Dudek H, Datta SR, Franke TF et al (1997) Regulation of neuronal survival by the serine-threonine protein kinase Akt. Science 275:661-664

27. Gajewski TF, Thompson CB (1996) Apoptosis meets signal transduction: Elimination of a BAD influence. Cell 87:589-592

28. Párrizas M, Le Roith D (1997) Insulin-like growth factor-I inhibition of apoptosis is associated with increased expression of the bcl-xl gene products. Endocrinology 138:1355-1358

29. Singleton JR, Dixit VM, Feldman EL (1996) Type I insulin-like growth factor receptor activation regulates apoptotic proteins. J Biol Chem 271:31791-31794

30. Jung Y-K, Miura M, Yuan J (1996) Suppression of interleukin-1β-converting enzyme-mediated cell death by insulin-like growth factor. J Biol Chem 271:5112-5117

31. Sell C, Baserga R, Rubin R (1995) Insulin-like growth factor-I (IGF-I) and the IGF-I receptor prevent etoposide-induced apoptosis. Cancer Res 55:303-306

32. Rodríguez-Tarduchy G, Collins MKL, García I, López-Rivas A (1992) Insulin-like growth factor 1 inhibits apoptosis in IL-3 dependent hemopoietic cells. J Immunol 149:535-540

33. Matthews CC, Feldman EL (1996) Insulin-like growth factor-1 rescues SH-SY5Y human neuroblastoma cells from hyperosmotic induced programmed cell death. J Cell Physiol 166:323-331

34. Werner H, Shen-orr Z, Rauscher FJI, Morris JF, Roberts CTJ, LeRoith D (1995) Inhibition of cellular proliferation by the Wilm's tumor suppressor WT1 is associated with suppression of insulin-like growth factor I receptor gene expression. Mol Cell Biol 15:3516-3522

35. Werner H, Karnieli E, Rauscher FJI, LeRoith D (1996) Wild-type and mutant p53 differentially regulate transcription of the insulin-like growth factor-I receptor gene. Proc Natl Acad Sci USA 93:8318-8323

36. Hernández-Sánchez C, Werner H, Roberts CTJ et al (1997) Differential regulation of insulin-like growth factor (IGF-I) receptor gene expression by IGF-I and basic fibroblast growth factor. J Biol Chem 272:4663-4670

IGF-I in Neuronal Differentiation and Neuroprotection

K. A. SULLIVAN[1], B. KIM[2], J. W. RUSSELL[2], E. L. FELDMAN[2]

Introduction

Insulin-like growth factors I and II (IGF-I and IGF-II) are peptide growth factors structurally related to insulin [1, 2]. Both IGF-I and IGF-II exert mitogenic and metabolic effects and influence differentiation in many cell types [3-6]. IGF-I and IGF-II are polypeptides essential for normal fetal, neonatal and pubertal growth [1, 2]. IGFs are present in a variety of tissues including muscle, lung, liver, kidney and brain during development and in the adult animal. Secreted IGFs may act as endocrine growth factors while locally synthesized peptides may serve autocrine/paracrine roles. Expression of IGFs is developmentally regulated in all species studied to date [7-15]. IGFs are abundant during fetal development [16-18], but there is a rapid decrease in IGF expression during the postnatal period [19, 20]. In the developing rat, IGFs are most abundant in neural crest derivatives, brain, choroid plexus, leptomeninges and spinal cord [16-18, 21]; similarly, in human embryogenesis, IGFs are present at high levels in fetal brain and spinal cord [21, 22]. IGFs share many important neurotrophic properties with nerve growth factor (NGF), the prototypic trophic factor [23, 24]. IGFs have neurotrophic actions in sensory [25], sympathetic [25, 26] and motor neurons [25], and are presently the only known neurotrophic factors in nerve and muscle capable of supporting both sensory and motor nerve regeneration in adult animals [27-32].

In the nervous system, IGF and IGF receptor are highly expressed during early fetal development, suggesting a role for these factors in synaptogenesis and myelination [1, 2, 14, 16, 33]. IGF-I mRNA is expressed in several brain regions during development [34-37]; expression is highest during late embryogenesis and early postpartum. IGF-I mRNA has been localized by in situ hybridization to Purkinje cells of the cerebellum, projection neurons of the cerebellar nuclei, ganglion cells of the retina and interneurons of the hippocampus and neocortex [34]. However, IGF-I mRNA expression is highest in developing cerebellum, midbrain and olfactory bulb [37, 38]. Developmental patterns of IGF-I expression also exhibit regional variability [39]. In cortex and hypothala-

Departments of Internal Medicine[1] and Neurology[2], University of Michigan, Ann Arbor, Michigan 48109 USA

mus, IGF-I mRNA levels peak at postnatal days 8 and 13, while in olfactory bulb levels are highest at day P21 and then steadily decrease [39].

IGF-I expression declines with adulthood in most tissues, however immunoreactive IGF-I has been detected in adult central nervous system (CNS) and in neurons and Schwann cells of adult autonomic and peripheral nervous systems [37, 40-42]. In humans, IGF-I mRNA and protein are present in fetal and adult brain, and IGF-I protein is present in cerebrospinal fluid [40, 43, 44]. In the adult rodent brain the same pattern of IGF-I mRNA distribution is observed; however, levels are diminished compared to those found in perinatal and young animal brains. The distinct developmental pattern of IGF expression in the nervous system supports the hypothesis that IGF stimulates neuronal and glial cell growth. In the central nervous system, IGF increases myelin production [45-47], stimulates DNA synthesis [48] and induces a catecholaminergic phenotype in chick neural crest cells [49]. Transgenic mice overexpressing IGF-I demonstrate increased brain size due to both increased neuronal size and number as well as increased myelination [50-52].

The biological actions of the IGFs are mediated by the type I IGF receptor (IGF-IR), a tyrosine kinase receptor. Like the IGFs, IGF-IR is expressed at the RNA and protein levels during fetal development of the brain, spinal cord and spinal ganglia [53-58]. IGF-IR expression reflects that of IGF-I during development. IGF-IR levels are highest during late embryogenesis and decline to adult levels soon after birth [19, 59]. Insulin receptors share a similar developmental pattern but levels remain somewhat higher than those of IGF-IR [19]. The anatomical distribution of IGF-IR is also closely related to that of IGF-I. Areas that exhibit high levels of [^{125}I]IGF-I binding include the olfactory bulb, cerebellum, cortex, choroid plexus and hippocampus [59-61].

Activation of IGF-IR results in tyrosine phosphorylation of a docking molecule, the insulin-receptor substrate-1 (IRS-1) [62]. IRS-1 is highly conserved between species [63] and is rapidly tyrosine phosphorylated in cells upon IGF-I treatment [62]. IRS-1 contains 21 potential tyrosine phosphorylation sites which create binding sites for SH-2 domain-containing proteins [63, 64], including the p85α-subunit of phosphatidylinositol-3 kinase (PI-3K), growth factor receptor bound-2 protein (GRB2), Syp, Nck and Crk [62-64]. GRB2 couples to the guanyl nucleotide exchange factor Sos, which in turn activates the Ras pathway where phosphorylation of c-Raf1 activates downstream protein kinases MAP kinase kinase 1 (also known as MEK or MKK1) or MAP kinase kinase 2 (MKK2). MKK1 and 2 activate two members of the MAP kinase family, ERK1 and ERK2, leading to activation and translocation of ERK1 and/or ERK2 to the nucleus; in the nucleus, the ERKs phosphorylate transcription factors including c-Fos, c-Jun, and c-Myc. This signaling cascade is activated by growth factors and is important for cellular growth and mitogenesis [62]. In contrast, phosphorylation and activation of PI-3K results in production of multi-phosphorylated forms of phosphatidylinositides which activate protein kinase C, along with a variety of other, more poorly characterized downstream targets [62, 65, 66]. This pathway involving PI-3K appears primarily to mediate growth factor-dependent motility and survival [67].

We believe the functions of IGFs are essential to normal nervous system growth and development. In our work, we use in vitro model systems of developing neurons to understand IGF action. SH-SY5Y human neuroblastoma cells provide a well-characterized model of neuronal growth to examine the role of IGFs in neuronal differentiation and survival [68-71]. Ultrastructurally, these cells resemble developing neurons, extend neuritic processes [72], and express functional cholinergic receptors [73] and voltage-gated Na^+, K^+, and Ca^{2+} channels [73-75]. Our data strongly suggest that IGFs and IGF-IR are essential for *initial growth cone motility*, as well as *long-term neurite outgrowth* and *protection against neuronal apoptosis*. In this review, we will examine each of these IGF-mediated events in SH-SY5Y cells.

IGF-I and Neuronal Motility

Growth cones are the highly motile tips of growing neurites. As they direct and guide neurite extension, growth cones respond to both internal and external cues. IGF-IR is abundantly expressed on growth cone membranes, suggesting that IGF-I is an important external cue for growth cone advancement (Fig.1). Addition of IGF-I results in immediate reorganization of actin filaments and the formation of membrane ruffles along the leading edge of the growth cone [67, 76]. As seen in Fig. 2, IGF-I-treated SH-SY5Y cells have a distinct, organized

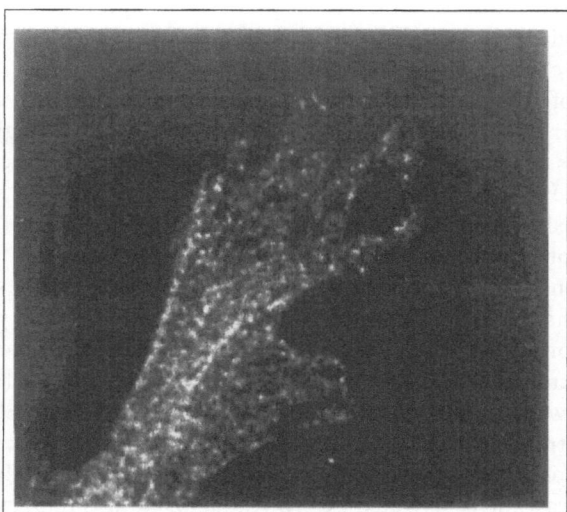

Fig. 1. Rat dorsal root ganglion (DRG) growth cones express IGF-I receptor. Dissociated E15 rat DRG neurons were cultured for 48 h, fixed in 4% paraformaldehyde and permeabilized. The neurons were then incubated in 10 µg/ml chicken IGF-IR IgY polyclonal antibody (Upstate Biotechnology) for 12 h, followed by 7.5 µg/ml goat anti-chicken secondary antibody and 50 µg/ml avidin-fluorescein (from Russel JW, Windebank AJ, Feldman EL (1998) Insulin-like growth factor-I prevents apoptosis in sensory neurons - in press)

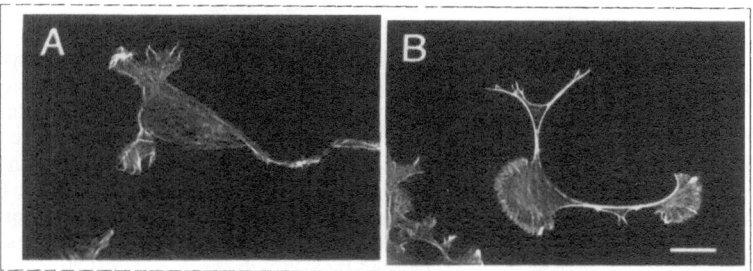

Fig. 2a, b. Organization of actin filaments in SH-SY5Y cells. Serum-starved SH-SY5Y cells were treated for 30 min with Dulbecco's modified Eagle's medium (DMEM) containing no addition (a) or 10 nM IGF-I (b). Actin filaments were localized by staining cells with rhodamine-phalloidin. Results are representative of four independent experiments. (From [76]). *Bar*, 10 μm

meshwork of actin at the lamellipodial edges of growth cones. Scanning electron micrographs (Fig. 3) highlight IGF-I-mediated ruffling, lamellipodial formation and protrusion of growth cone membranes. As growth cones advance, they adhere to specific extracellular matrix molecules and form focal adhesions by tyrosine phosphorylation of two proteins: paxillin and focal adhesion kinase (FAK) [67,76-78]. IGF-I activates FAK and paxillin (Fig. 4) which are concen-

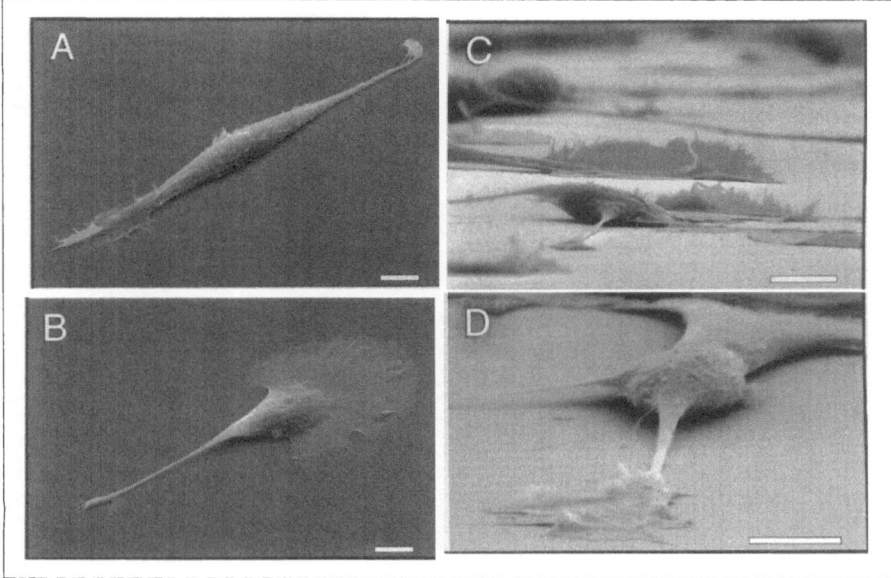

Fig. 3a-d. Characterization of SH-SY5Y cell morphology by scanning electron microscopy. Serum-starved SH-SY5Y cells were treated for 30 min with DMEM containing no addition (a) or 10 nM IGF-I (b-d). (From [76]). *Bars*, 10 μm

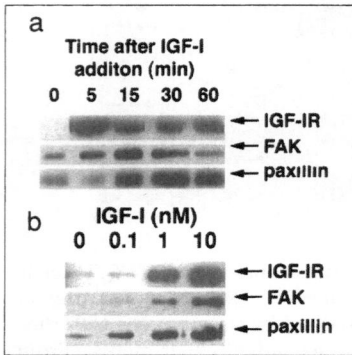

a

Time after IGF-I additon (min)

0   5   15   30   60

←— IGF-IR
←— FAK
←— paxillin

b

IGF-I (nM)

0   0.1   1   10

←— IGF-IR
←— FAK
←— paxillin

Fig. 4a, b. IGF-I-stimulated tyrosine phosphorylation of FAK, paxillin, and IGF-IR. Serum-starved SH-SY5Y cells were treated with DMEM containing IGF-I in the specified conditions. Cells were lysed and proteins were immunoprecipitated with antibodies specific to IGF-IR, FAK, or paxillin. Equal amounts of total cellular protein were used for each condition in an experiment. Isolated proteins were separated by SDS-polyacrylamide gel electrophoresis (SDS-PAGE), transferred to nitrocellulose, and analyzed by anti-phosphotyrosine immunoblotting. **a** Time course of IGF-I-stimulated tyrosine phorphorylation. SH-SY5Y cells were treated with DMEM containing 10 nM IGF-I for 0-60 min. The 0 time point indicates cells treated with DMEM alone. **b** Concentration response of IGF-I-stimulated tyrosine phosphorylation. SH-SY5Y cells were treated for 30 min with DMEM containing 0-10 nM IGF-I. Results are representative of four independent experiments. (From [76])

trated in the lamellipodial membrane of growth cones (Fig. 5). The PI-3K arm of the IGF-IR signalling pathway appears more involved in IGF-I-mediated lamellipodial formation and activation of focal adhesions, and may involve activation of the small G protein, Rac [67]. Further studies are required to confirm this concept (Fig. 6).

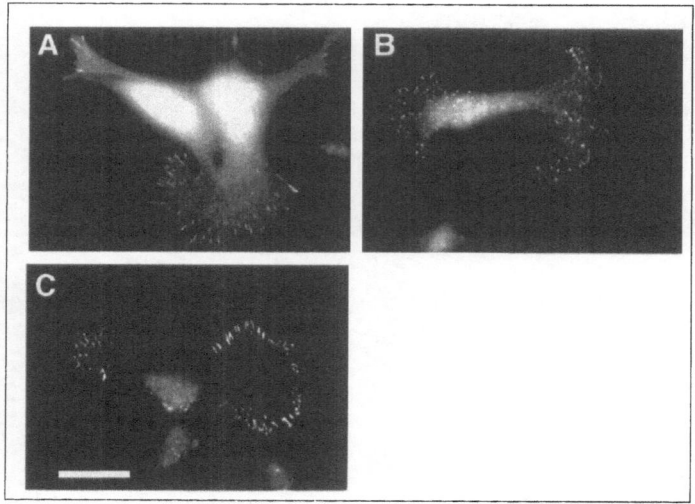

Fig. 5a-c. Localization of FAK, paxillin, and phosphotyrosine in IGF-I-treated SH-SY5Y cells. Serum-starved SH-SY5Y cells were treated for 30 min with DMEM containing 10 nM IGF-I. Cells were then stained for FAK (**a**), paxillin (**b**), or phosphotyrosine (**c**). Results are representative of four independent experiments. (From [76]). *Bar*, 25 μm

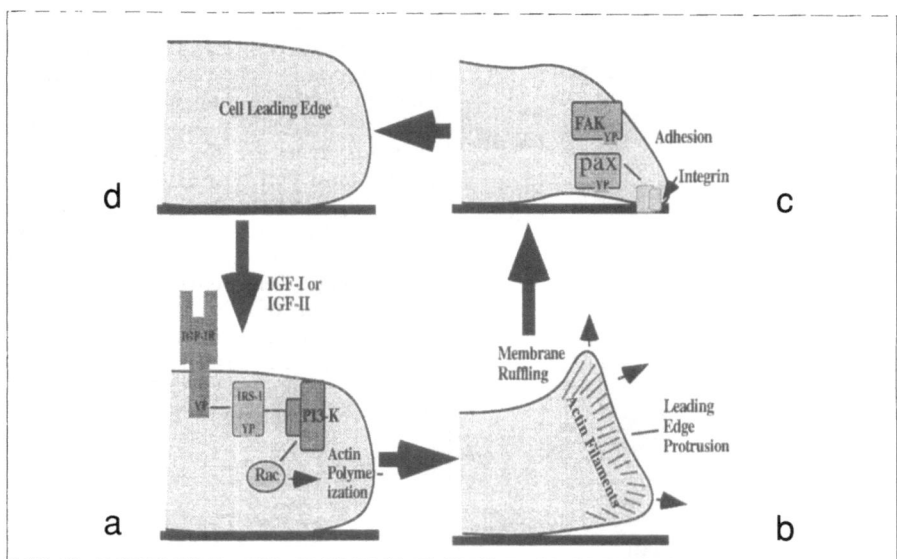

Fig. 6a-d. Potential sequence of events by which IGFs promote cell motility. **a** IGFs bind to IGF-IR, stimulating receptor autophosphorylation, IRS-1 phosphorylation, and activation of PI-3 kinase. This may result in the activation of Rac, which, in turn, promotes actin polymerization. **b** Polymerization of actin leads to membrane ruffling and protrusion of the leading edge. **c** Protruding membranes adhere to the extracellular matrix via integrins and are stabilized by FAK and paxillintyrosine phosphorylation. FAK and paxillintyrosine phosphorylation and associated integrin-extracellular matrix adhesion may require activation of PI-3 kinase. **d** Repetition of the cycle, coupled with release of old adhesions, allows continued lamellipodial advance and eventual cell migration or growth cone translocation. *YP*, sites of tyrosine phosphorylation. (From [67])

IGF-I and Long-term Neurite Outgrowth

We [70, 72] and others [79-82] have shown that IGF-I treatment also results in vigorous long-term neurite outgrowth. We have begun to characterize the downstream signaling pathways required for IGF-I-mediated neurite outgrowth and to address whether this long-term IGF-I effect is separable from IGF-I's short-term effects on growth cone motility. In preliminary experiments, we found that IGF-I induced a concentration-dependent increase of tyrosine phosphorylation of the IGF-IR β-subunit and of ERK2 for at least 24 h in SH-SY5Y cells [83] (Fig. 7A). Activation of IGF-IR and ERK2 correlated with IGF-mediated neurite outgrowth in neuroblastoma cells (Fig. 7B). When ERK2 activation was blocked by PD98059, a selective MEK inhibitor, we observed a concentration-dependent decrease in the IGF-I-stimulated tyrosine phosphorylation of ERK2 (Fig. 8A) and in its ability to phosphorylate an Elk-1 fusion protein (Fig. 8B) without affecting IGF-IR tyrosine phosphorylation. In parallel, PD98059 treatment also inhibited IGF-I-mediated increases in GAP-43 (the most abundant neuron-specific protein in neuronal growth cones) (Fig. 8C) and IGF-I-stimulated neurite outgrowth (Fig. 8D).

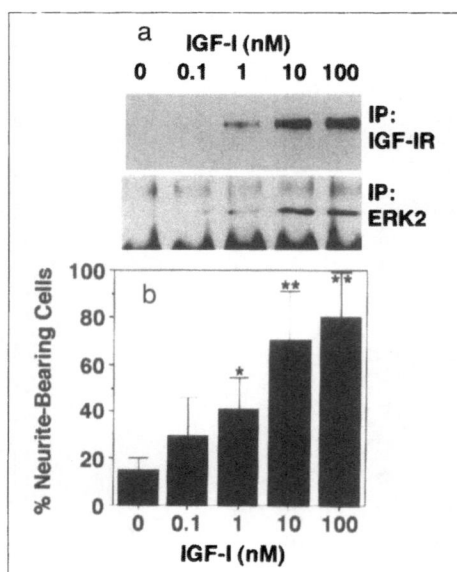

Fig. 7a, b. Concentration dependence of IGF-I-stimulated IGF-IR and ERK2 tyrosine phosphorylation parallels increased neurite outgrowth. **a** Serum-starved SH-SY5Y cells were treated with increasing concentrations of IGF-I for 30 min. Equal amounts of cell lysates (500 µg) were immunoprecipitated with anti-IGF-IR or anti-ERK2 antibody before analysis by SDS-PAGE and anti-phosphotyrosine western blotting. **b** Cells were treated with indicated amounts of IGF-I for 24 h and neurite-bearing cells were scored. Results are mean ± SEM of at least 3 separate observations. *$P < 0.005$, and **$P < 0.001$ (by independent Student's t test). (From [83])

Collectively, these results suggest that IGF-I stimulates long-term neurite outgrowth by ERK activation and support previous reports from our laboratory [70, 76, 84, 85] and from others [79-82, 86-88] indicating that IGF-I mediates neuronal differentiation.

IGF-I is a Neuroprotective Agent

Apoptosis, also referred to as programmed cell death (PCD), is a ubiquitous phenomenon essential for normal development and integral to the pathogenesis of many diseases [89]. In many cell types, PCD follows the withdrawal of a required growth factor or the introduction of a noxious stimulus [90-94]. PCD, then, can be thought of as a "default" program that all cells are poised to enter unless continually restrained by selective factors [95, 96]. Although the mechanism of mammalian PCD is not understood, comparison with nematode cell death regulators has identified two classes of death effectors: (1) a family of proto-oncogenes which includes genes encoding Bcl-2, Bcl-x_L and Bax [97], and (2) a family of cysteine proteases designated as interleukin-1β converting enzyme-like molecules [98, 99].

Bcl Family

Bcl-2 is a protein located in mitochondrial, endoplasmic reticular and perinuclear membranes [100] which suppresses naturally occuring cell death [95, 97, 101]. Bcl-x_L appears to function in a manner similar to Bcl-2, while Bcl-x_S

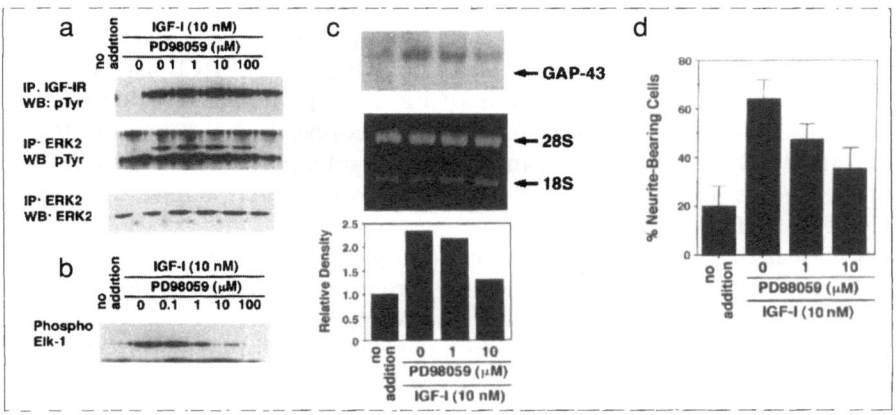

Fig. 8a-d. The MEK inhibitor PD98059 blocks IGF-I-induced ERK2 activation, GAP-43 gene expression and neurite outgrowth. **a** Anti-phosphotyrosine western blotting. Serum-starved SH-SY5Y cells were treated with increasing concentrations of PD98059 for 1 h prior to a 30 min incubation with 10 nM IGF-I. Cell lysates (500 µg) were immunoprecipitated (*IP*) with anti-IGF-IR or anti-ERK2 antibodies followed by SDS-PAGE and anti-phosphotyrosine or anti-ERK2 western blotting (*WB*). Results are representative of at least 3 separate experiments. **b** Effect of PD98059 on MAP kinase activity. Equal amounts of cell lysate were immunoprecipitated with an antibody specific to phosphorylated MAP kinase. Immunoprecipitated MAP kinase was incubated with 1 µg Elk-1 fusion protein in kinase buffer (25 mM Tris, pH 7.5, 5 mM β-glycerolphosphate, 2 mM dithiothreitol, 0.1 mM Na$_3$VO$_4$, and 10 mM MgCl$_2$). The mixture was subjected to SDS-PAGE and analyzed by western blotting using anti-phosphorylated Elk-1 (*Phospho Elk-1*). **c** Serum-starved cells were treated with 10 nM IGF-I in the presence of 0-10 µM PD98059. Control cells were treated with 0.1% DMSO alone. After 24 h, total RNA was isolated from all samples. *Top*, Northern blot analysis using 32P-labeled cDNA probes for *GAP-43*. *Middle*, Ethidium bromide staining of the agarose gels. *Bottom*, Relative values from densitometric analyses of autoradiographs. Results are the representative of 3 separate experiments. **d** Serum-starved SH-SY5Y cells were treated with 10 nM IGF-I for 24 h in the presence of 0-10 µM PD98059. Control cells were treated with 0.1% DMSO alone. After 24 h, neurite-bearing cells were scored. Results are mean + SEM of at least 3 separate observations. $P < 0.001$ (by independent Student's t test) compared to the cells treated with 10 nM IGF-I only. (From [83])

blocks Bcl-2 and Bcl-x$_L$ functions. Bcl-2 is highly expressed in the developing central and peripheral nervous systems [102]. With maturation of the CNS, Bcl-2 appears to be replaced by Bcl-x$_L$ [102, 103], while the mature peripheral nervous system continues to express high levels of Bcl-2 [102]. Overexpression or direct microinjection of Bcl-2 protects neurons against apoptosis [104-107] while targeted disruption of *Bcl-x$_L$* gene during embryogenesis results in massive neuronal death [108].

ICE-like Proteases: Death Enhancers

Interleukin-1β converting enzyme (ICE) is a cysteine protease that activates pro-interleukin-1β by cleavage at aspartate residues [98, 99]. Blocking ced-

3/ICE-like protease activity prevents PCD in many cell types [109-111], confirming that proteolytic cleavage of specific death substrates is a critical biochemical event in early PCD. At least seven homologs of ced-3/ICE-like protease have been identified, including Yama/CPP32/apopain [112-114] and ICE-LAP3/Mch3/CMH-1 [115]. Phylogenetic analysis reveals that Yama and ICE-LAP3 are closely related to ced-3, and compose a subfamily whose members are synthesized as pro-enzymes and processed to form active heterodimeric enzymes [116, 117].

It is clear that Bcl-2 and Bcl-x$_L$ function upstream of Yama and ICE-LAP3 [117]. Once apoptotic stimuli overcome the "protection" provided by the Bcl proteins, Yama and/or ICE-LAP3 are activated; in turn, these proteases cleave a death substrate, the 116 kDa nuclear protein poly(ADP-ribose) polymerase (PARP) [118, 119] to yield an 85 kDa apoptotic fragment [118], which is present in virtually every form of PCD examined [118, 120-122]. The exact role of these death substrates in the execution phase of apoptosis is a current area of investigation. Mammalian cells likely possess several ICE-like proteases which may each cleave one or more death substrates to execute an apoptotic pathway [116, 117].

IGF-I and Apoptosis

There is strong evidence that IGF-I treatment blocks neuronal apoptosis [123-126]. IGF-I rescues cerebellar neurons from ion-coupled apoptosis [93] and reduces PCD in human erythroid progenitor cells [127]. The removal of IGF-I initiates PCD in cultured granule neurons [93] and PC12 cells [90], while transfection with a plasmid constitutively expressing the complete human IGF-IR cDNA allows autonomous growth of neurons [124]. While IGF-IR overexpression enhances cell viability, antisense strategies to block IGF-IR expression induce cellular growth arrest [128-131]. PCD is a highly regulated process with control points at transcriptional, translational and post-translational levels [117]. We are interested in understanding at which control point (or points) does IGF-IR activation interrupt a death cascade in neurons stimulated to apoptosis. Hyperosmolar stress is a potent apoptotic stimulus for neural cells [123, 124, 126]. Greater than 60% of SH-SY5Y cells undergo PCD (as quantitated by DNA fragmentation analysis and flow cytometry) within 24 h after exposure to 300 mM mannitol [124, 126]. In this paradigm, IGF-I rescues neurons from osmotically induced PCD and decreases by more than 10-fold the number of cells induced to PCD.

We used immunoblot analysis of cellular lysates to probe for changes in total cellular pools of Bcl-2, Bcl-x$_L$ and Bax prior to and 24 h following treatment of SH-SY5Y cells with 300 mM mannitol with or without 10 nM IGF-II. Twenty-four hours following mannitol treatment there was a clear decrease in total cellular Bcl-2 (as a fraction of total cellular protein) which was prevented by addition of IGF (Fig. 9A). The cellular Bcl-x$_L$ pool was also reduced, although to a lesser degree. Following 24 h of mannitol treatment, total cellular Bax was not altered appreciably, though larger mol. wt. forms were apparent on immunoblot analysis. Treatment with IGF-II prevented appearance of these larger forms, which may represent dimerization or binding of Bax with Bcl-2 or Bcl-x_L [125].

We have also examined SHEP neuroblastoma cells transfected with human IGF-IR cDNA in either correct orientation (FB+2, stably increasing cell surface IGF-IR abundance 5-15 fold), or reverse orientation (FC-4) as a control. Total cellular pools of Bcl proteins in FB+2 and FC-4 during log phase growth were compared. Overexpression of IGF-IR in FB+2 resulted in increased total cellular pool of Bcl-x_L compared to the control transfectant FC-4 (Fig. 10). Bax and Bcl-2 concentrations were similar for the two transfectants. These preliminary studies suggest a potential long-term regulation of Bcl proteins by IGF-IR activation.

During propogation of a death signal, the 32 kD proform of the ICE-like protease Yama and the 35 kD proform of ICE/LAP3 are proteolytically cleaved to active forms. High mannitol treatment rapidly induced conversion of proYama (32 kD) to active Yama (17 and 24 kD forms) in SH-SY5Y cells (Fig. 11A). The 17 kD Yama fragment appeared in cell lysates within 6 h of exposure to 300 mM mannitol. IGF-II prevented proteolytic activation of Yama and ICE/LAP3 (Fig. 11B), an effect which correlates with our previous finding that IGF-I reduced 10-fold the number of cells subjected to mannitol-induced DNA fragmentation at 24 h [124, 126].

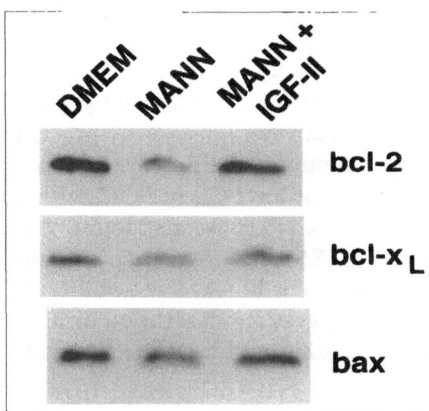

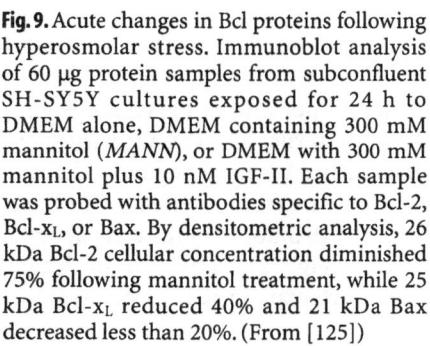

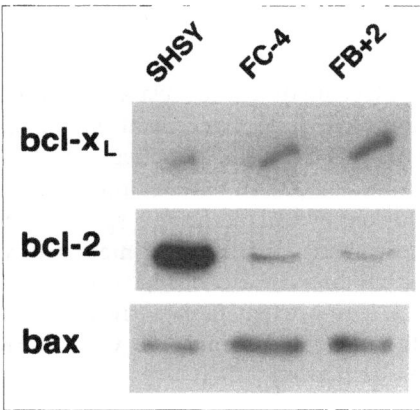

Fig. 9. Acute changes in Bcl proteins following hyperosmolar stress. Immunoblot analysis of 60 µg protein samples from subconfluent SH-SY5Y cultures exposed for 24 h to DMEM alone, DMEM containing 300 mM mannitol (*MANN*), or DMEM with 300 mM mannitol plus 10 nM IGF-II. Each sample was probed with antibodies specific to Bcl-2, Bcl-x_L, or Bax. By densitometric analysis, 26 kDa Bcl-2 cellular concentration diminished 75% following mannitol treatment, while 25 kDa Bcl-x_L reduced 40% and 21 kDa Bax decreased less than 20%. (From [125])

Fig. 10. Effects of chronically increased IGF-IR abundance on cellular concentrations of Bcl proteins. SH-SY5Y cells, control SHEP transfectant FC-4, or SHEP/IGF-IR transfectant FB+2 (which expresses 6-fold more cell surface IGF-IR than does FC-4) were grown to 90% confluence in DMEM with 10% calf serum. Total protein lysates (60 µg) were separated by SDS-PAGE and subjected to immunoblot analysis using antibodies specific to Bcl-x_L, Bcl-2 or Bax. Results are representative of three experiments. (From [125])

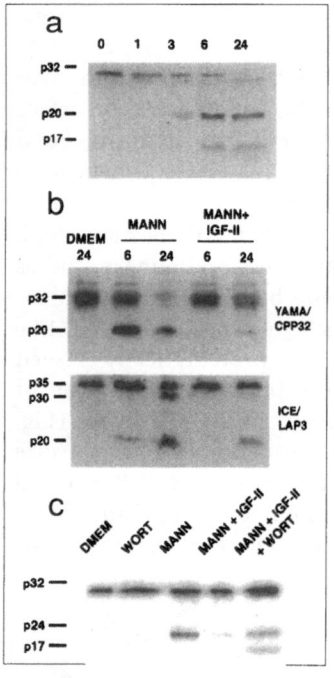

Fig. 11a-c. Effects of IGF-IR activation on ICE-like protease activity. a SH-SY5Y cells were exposed to 300 mM mannitol for the indicated times (h). Total protein lysates were size-fractionated by SDS-PAGE and immunoblotted with antibody to p17 Yama/CPP32. The 17 and 24 kDa active, proteolytic fragments of Yama appeared within 3 h of exposure, reaching maximum by 6 h. b Exogenous IGF-II retarded the proteolytic processing of Yama and ICE/LAP3. SH-SY5Y cells were exposed for the indicated times (h) to DMEM or to DMEM containing 300 mM mannitol (*MANN*) alone or with 10 nM IGF-II (*MANN + IGF-II*). PAGE-separated proteins were immunoblotted with antibody to p17 Yama/CPP32 or to p20 ICE/LAP3. c SH-SY5Y cells were exposed for 6 h to PI-3K inhibitor wortmannin (*WORT*, 100 nM). Wortmannin blocked the ability of IGF-II to inhibit Yama processing. Results are representative of three experiments. (From [125])

Recent studies suggest a link between IGF-I activation of PI-3K and protection from PCD. Concentrations of insulin which activate IGF-IR [62] prevent PCD in PC12 cells by activating PI-3K, independently of the Ras-MAP-kinase pathway [132]. In parallel, the ability of insulin to prevent PCD in PC12 cells is blocked by wortmannin, a specific inhibitor of PI-3K [132]. We also found that wortmannin blocked IGF-mediated rescue of SH-SY5Y cells from hyperosmolar-mediated PCD. In Fig. 11C, wortmannin treatment blocked the ability of IGF-II to prevent Yama activation. These results suggest that activation of IGF-IR by IGF-II prevents PCD via a PI-3K signaling pathway, although more studies are needed [124].

Summary

IGF-I and IGF-IR are expressed in the central and peripheral nervous systems during developmental and exhibit cell-specific patterns. IGF-I is a potent neurotrophic factor for both sensory and motor neurons. We have begun to characterize the mechanisms which underlie IGF-I's neurotrophic effects. We have found that IGF-I enhances growth cone motility, promotes long-term neurite outgrowth and protects neurons from apoptosis (Fig. 12). Activation of different IGF-IR signaling cascades by IGF-I may, in part, explain IGF-I's pleotrophic effects.

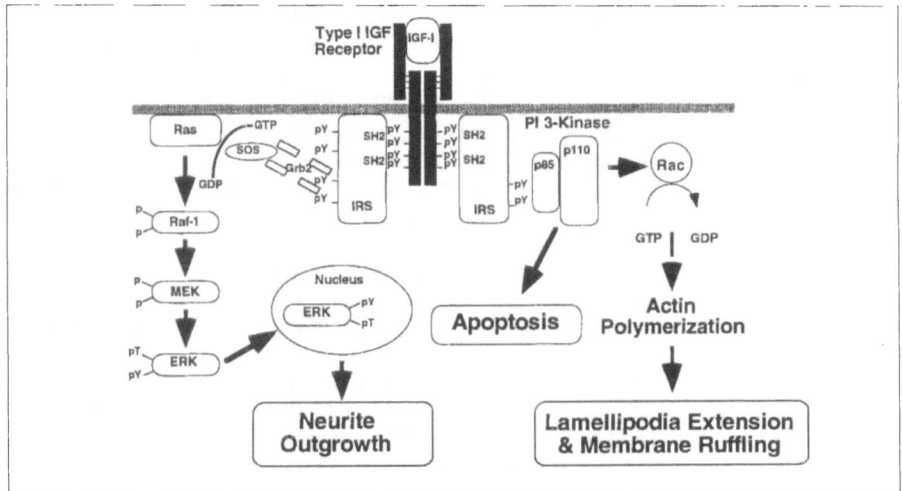

Fig. 12. IGF-I mediates neuronal differentiation and survival. Proposed pathways for IGF-I-mediated neurite outgrowth, protection against apoptosis and changes in growth cone morphology

Acknowledgements

This work was supported by NIH grants R29 NS32843 (ELF), K08 NS01938 (JWR) and grants from the American Diabetes Association, Juvenile Diabetes Foundation International and the Muscular Dystrophy Association. The authors would like to thank Drs. Phillip Leventhal (supported by 1F32 NS09912) and J. Robinson Singleton for their contributions, Judy Boldt for expert secretarial assistance, and James Beals for help with digital image processing.

References

1. Daughaday WH, Rotwein P (1989) Insulin-like growth factor I and II. Peptide, messenger ribonucleic acid and gene structures, serum, and tissue concentrations. Endocr Rev 10(1):68-91
2. Sara VR, Hall K (1990) Insulin-like growth factors and their binding proteins. Physiol Rev 70:591-614
3. Tollefsen SE, Lajara R, McCusker RH, Clemmons DR, Rotwein P (1989) Insulin-like growth factors (IGF) in muscle development. J Biol Chem 264(23):13810-13817
4. Levy MJ, Hernandez ER, Adashi EY, Stillman RJ, Roberts CT Jr, LeRoith D (1992) Expression of the insulin-like growth factor (IGF)-I and -II and the IGF-I and -II receptor genes during postnatal development of the rat ovary. Endocrinology 131:1202-1206
5. Nyman T, Pekonen F (1993) The expression of insulin-like growth factors and their binding proteins in normal human lymphocytes. Acta Endocrinol 128:168-172

6. Rosen KM, Wentworth BM, Rosenthal N, Villa-Komaroff L (1993) Specific, temporally regulated expression of the insulin-like growth factor II gene during muscle cell differentiation. Endocrinology 133:474-481

7. Moses AC, Nissley SP, Short PA, Rechler MM, White RM, Knight AB, Higa OZ (1980) Increased levels of multiplication-stimulating activity, an insulin-like growth factor, in fetal rat serum. Proc Natl Acad Sci USA 77(6):3649-3653

8. Brown AL, Graham DE, Nissley SP, Hill DJ, Strain AJ, Rechler MM (1986) Developmental regulation of insulin-like growth factor II mRNA in different rat tissues. J Biol Chem 261(28):13144-13150

9. Graham DE, Rechler MM, Brown AL, Frunzio R, Romanus JA, Bruni CB, Whitfield HJ, Nessley SP, Seelig S, Berry S (1986) Coordinate developmental regulation of high and low molecular weight mRNAs for rat insulin-like growth factor II. Proc Natl Acad Sci USA 83:4519-4523

10. Lund PK, Moats-Staats BM, Hynes MA, Simmons JG, Jansen M, D'Ercole AJ, Van Wyk JJ (1986) Somatomedin-C/insulin-like growth factor-I and insulin-like growth factor-II mRNAs in rat fetal and adult tissues. J Biol Chem 261(3):14539-14544

11. Kukuchi K, Buonomo FC, Kajimoto Y, Rotwein P (1991) Expression of insulin-like growth factor-I during chicken development. Endocrinology 128(3):1323-1328

12. Lee CY, Bazer FW, Etherton TD, Simmen FA (1991) Ontogeny of insulin-like growth factors (IGF-I and IGF-II) and IGF-binding proteins in porcine serum during fetal and postnatal development. Endocrinology 128:2336-2344

13. Lee CY, Chung CS, Simmen FA (1993) Ontogeny of the porcine insulin-like growth factor system. Mol Cell Endocrinol 93:71-80

14. Liu F, Powell DR, Styne DM, Hintz RL (1991) Insulin-like growth factors (IGFs) and IGF-binding proteins in the developing rhesus monkey. J Clin Endocrinol Metab 72:905-911

15. Werner H, Woloschak M, Adamo M, Shen-Orr Z, Roberts CT, LeRoith D (1989) Developmental regulation of the rat insulin-like growth factor I receptor gene. Proc Natl Acad Sci USA 86:7451-7455

16. Beck F, Samani NJ, Byrne S, Morgan K, Gebhard R, Brammar WJ (1988) Histochemical localization of IGF-I and IGF-II mRNA in the rat between birth and adulthood. Development 104:29-39

17. Stylianopoulou F, Herbert J, Soares MB, Efstratiadis A (1988) Expression of the insulin-like growth factor II gene in the choroid plexus and the leptomeninges of the adult rat central nervous system. Proc Natl Acad Sci USA 85:141-145

18. Lee JE, Pintar J, Efstratiadis A (1990) Pattern of the insulin-like growth factor II gene expression during early mouse embryogenesis. Development 110:151-159

19. Van Evercooren AB, Olichon-Berthe C (1991) Expression of IGF-I and insulin receptor genes in the rat central nervous system: a developmental, regional, and cellular analysis. J Neurosci Res 28:244-253

20. Adem A, Jossan SS, d'Argy R, Gillberg PG, Nordberg A, Winblad B, Sara V (1989) Insulin-like growth factor 1 (IGF-1) receptors in the human brain: quantitative autoradiographic localization. Brain Res 503:299-303

21. Sullivan KA, Feldman EL (1994) Immunohistochemical localization of insulin-like growth factor II and insulin-like growth factor binding protein-2 during development in the rat. Endocrinology 135:540-547

22. Sara VR, Carlsson-Skwirut C, Andersson C, Hall E, Sjogren B, Holmgren A, Jornval H (1986) Characterization of somatomedins from human fetal brain: Identification of a variant form of insulin-like growth factor I. Proc Natl Acad Sci USA 83:4904-4907

23. Bothwell M (1995) Functional interactions of neurotrophins and neurotrophin receptors. Annu Rev Neurosci 18:223-253

24. Parada LF, Tsoulfas P, Tessarollo L, Blair J, Reid SW, Soppet D (1992) The Trk family of tyrosine kinases: receptors for NGF-related neurotrophins. Cold Spring Harb Symp Quant Biol 57:43-51

25. Ishii DN, Glazner GW, Pu S-F (1994) Role of insulin-like growth factors in peripheral nerve regeneration. Pharmacol Ther 62:125-144

26. Zackenfels K, Oppenheim RW, Rohrer H (1995) Evidence for an important role of IGF-I and IGF-II for the early development of chick sympathetic neurons. Neuron 14:731-741

27. Houenou LJ, Li L, Lo AC, Yan Q, Oppenheim RW (1994) Naturally occurring and axotomy-induced motoneuron death and its prevention by neurotrophic agents: a comparison between chick and mouse. In: van Pelt J, Corner MA, Uylings HBM, Lopes da Silva FH (eds) Progress in brain research. Elsevier, Amsterdam, pp 217-226

28. Contreras PC, Steffler C, Yu EY, Callison K, Stong D, Vaught JL (1995) Systemic administration of rhIGF-I enhanced regeneration after sciatic nerve crush in mice. J Pharmacol Exp Ther 274:1443-1449

29. Glazner GW, Lupien S, Miller JA, Ishii DN (1993) Insulin-like growth factor II increases the rate of sciatic nerve regeneration in rats. Neuroscience 54:791-797

30. Ishii DN (1995) Implication of insulin-like growth factors in the pathogenesis of diabetic neuropathy. Brain Res Rev 20:47-67

31. Ishii D, Marsh D (1993) On the therapeutic potential for insulin-like growth factor use in motor neuron disease. Neurology 124:96-99

32. Lewis ME, Vaught JL, Neff NT, Grebow PE, Callison KV, Yu E, Contreras PC, Baldino F (1993) The potential of insulin-like growth factor-I as a therapeutic for the treatment of neuromuscular disorders. Ann N Y Acad Sci 692:201-208

33. Clemmons DR (1989) Structural and functional analysis of insulin-like growth factors. Br Med Bull 45(2):465 480

34. Lee W-H, Michels KM, Bondy CA (1993) Localization of insulin-like growth factor binding protein-2 messenger RNA during postnatal brain development: Correlation with insulin-like growth factors I and II. Neuroscience 53:251-265

35. Bondy CA (1991) Transient IGF-I gene expression during the maturation of functionally related central projection neurons. J Neurosci 11:3442-3455

36. Bondy C, Lee W-H (1993) Correlation between insulin-like growth factor (IGF)-binding protein 5 and IGF-I gene expression during brain development. J Neurosci 13:5092-5104

37. Rotwein P, Burgess SK, Milbrandt JD, Krause JE (1988) Differential expression of insulin-like growth factor genes in rat central nervous sytem. Proc Natl Acad Sci USA 85:265-269

38. Simmen FA, Simmen RCM (1991) Peptide growth factors and proto-oncogenes in mammalian conceptus development. Biol Reprod 44:1-5

39. Bach MA, Shen-Orr Z, Lowe WL Jr, Roberts CT, LeRoith D (1991) Insulin-like growth factor I mRNA levels are developmentally regulated in specific regions of the rat brain. Mol Brain Res 10:43-48

40. Haselbacher GK, Schwab ME, Pasi A, Humbel RE (1985) Insulin-like growth factor II (IGF II) in human brain: Regional distribution of IGF II and of higher molecular mass forms. Proc Natl Acad Sci USA 82:2153-2157

41. Hansson HA, Dahlin LB, Danielsen N, Fryklund L, Nachemson AK, Polleryd P, Rozell B, Skottner A, Stemme S, Lundborg G (1986) Evidence indicating trophic importance of IGF-I in regenerating peripheral nerves. Acta Physiol Scand 126:609-614

42. Garcia-Segura LM, Perez J, Pons S, Rejas MT, Torres-Aleman I (1991) Localization of insulin-like growth factor I (IGF-I)-like immunoreactivity in the developing and adult rat brain. Brain Res 560:167-174

43. Han VKM, Lund PK, Lee DC, D'Ercole AJ (1988) Expression of somatomedin/insulin-like growth factor messenger ribonucleic acids in the human fetus: identification, characterization, and tissue distribution. J Clin Endocrinol Metab 66:422-429

44. Backstrom M, Hall K, Sara V (1984) Somatomedin levels in cerebrospinal fluid from adults with pituitary disorders. Acta Endocrinol (Copenh) 107:171-178

45. Mozell RL, McMorris FA (1991) Insulin-like growth factor I stimulates oligodendrocyte development and myelination in rat brain aggregate cultures. J Neurosci Res 30:382-390

46. McMorris FA, Mozell RL, Carson MJ, Shinar Y, Meyer RD, Marchetti N (1993) Regulation of oligodendrocyte development and central nervous system myelination by insulin-like growth factors. Ann N Y Acad Sci 692:321-334

47. Carson MJ, Behringer RR, Brinster RL, McMorris FA (1993) Insulin-like growth factor I increases brain growth and central nervous system myelination in transgenic mice. Neuron 10:729-740

48. Lenoir D, Honegger P (1983) Insulin-like growth factor I (IGF I) stimulates DNA synthesis fetal rat brain cell cultures. Dev Brain Res 7:205-213

49. Nataf V, Monier S (1992) Effect of insulin and insulin-like growth factor I on the expression of the catecholaminergic phenotype by neural crest cells. Dev Brain Res 69:59-66

50. Morgan JI, Curran T (1991) Stimulus-transcription coupling in the nervous system: Involvement of the inducible proto-oncogenes fos and jun. Annu Rev Neurosci 14:421-451

51. Ye P, Carson J, D'Ercole AJ (1995) In vivo actions of insulin-like growth factor-I (IGF-I) on brain myelination: Studies of IGF-I and IGF binding protein-1 (IGFBP-1) transgenic mice. J Neurosci 15:7344-7356

52. Ye P, Carson J, D'Ercole AJ (1995) Insulin-like growth factor-I influences the initiation of myelination: Studies of the anterior commissure of transgenic mice. Neurosci Lett 201:235-238

53. Bondy C, Werner H, Roberts CT, LeRoith D (1992) Cellular pattern of type-I insulin-like growth factor receptor gene expression during maturation of the rat brain: Comparison with insulin-like growth factors I and II. Neuroscience 46:909-923

54. MacDonald RG (1991) Mannose-6-phosphate enhances cross-linking efficiency between insulin-like growth factor-II (IGF-II) and IGF-II/mannose-6-phosphate receptors in membranes. Endocrinology 128:413-421

55. Gammeltoft S, Haselbacher GK, Humbel RE, Fehlmann M, Van Obberghen E (1985) Two types of receptor for insulin-like growth factors in mammalian brain. EMBO J 4:3407-3412

56. Sklar MM, Thomas CL, Municchi G, Roberts CT, LeRoith D, Kiess W, Nissley P (1992) Developmental expression of rat insulin-like growth factor-II/mannose 6-phosphate receptor messenger ribonucleic acid. Endocrinology 130:3484-3491

57. Sklar MM, Kies W, Thomas CL, Nissley SP (1989) Developmental expression of the tissue insulin-like growth factor II/mannose 6-phosphate receptor in the rat. J Biol Chem 264:16733-16738

58. Bondy CA, Werner H, Roberts CT Jr, LeRoith D (1990) Cellular pattern of insulin-like growth factor-I (IGF-I) and type I IGF receptor gene expression in early organogenesis: comparison with IGF-II gene expression. Mol Endocrinol 4:1386-1398

59. Kar S, Chabot J-G, Quirion R (1993) Quantitative autoradiographic localization of [^{125}I]insulin-like growth factor I, [^{125}I]insulin-like growth factor II, and [^{125}I]insulin receptor binding sites in developing and adult rat brain. J Comp Neurol 333:375-397

60. Lesniak MA, Hill JM, Kiess W, Rojeski M, Pert CB, Roth J (1988) Receptors for insulin-

like growth factors I and II: autoradiographic localization in rat brain and comparison to receptors for insulin. Endocrinology 123 (4):2089-2099

61. Araujo DM, Lapchak PA, Collier B, Chabot J-G, Quirion R (1989) Insulin-like growth factor-1 (somatomedin-C) receptors in the rat brain: distribution and interaction with the hippocampal cholinergic system. Brain Res 484:130-138

62. De Meyts P, Wallach B, Christoffersen CT, Urso B, Gronskov K, Latus L-J, Yakushiji F, Ilondo MM, Shymko RM (1994) The insulin-like growth factor-I receptor. Structure, ligand-binding mechanism and signal transduction. Horm Res 42:152-169

63. White M, Kahn CR (1994) The insulin signaling system. J Biol Chem 269:1-4

64. Eck MJ, Dhe-Paganon S, Trub T, Nolte RT, Shoelson SE (1996) Structure of the IRS-1 PTB domain bound to the juxtamembrane region of the insulin receptor. Cell 85:695-705

65. Nishida E, Gotoh Y (1993) The MAP kinase cascade is essential for diverse signal transduction pathways. Trends Biochem Sci 18:128-131

66. Pelech SL, Sanghera JS (1992) Mitogen-activated protein kinases: versatile transducers for cell signaling. Trends Biochem Sci 17:233-238

67. Leventhal PS, Feldman EL (1997) Insulin-like growth factors as regulators of cell motility: signaling mechanisms. Trends Endocrinol Metab 8:1-6

68. Martin DM, Yee D, Carlson RO, Feldman EL (1992) Gene expression of the insulin-like growth factors and their receptors in human neuroblastoma cells. Mol Brain Res 15:241-246

69. Martin DM, Feldman EL (1993) Regulation of insulin-like growth factor-II expression and its role in autocrine growth of human neuroblastoma cells. J Cell Physiol 155:290-300

70. Sumantran VN, Feldman EL (1993) Insulin-like growth factor I regulates c-myc and GAP-43 messenger ribonucleic acid expression in SH-SY5Y human neuroblastoma cells. Endocrinology 132:2017-2023

71. Meghani MA, Martin DM, Singleton JR, Feldman EL (1993) Effects of serum and insulin-like growth factors on human neuroblastoma cell growth. Regul Pept 48:217-224

72. Feldman EL, Randolph AE (1991) Mannose 6-phosphate potentiates insulin-like growth factor II effects in cultured human neuroblastoma cells. Brain Res 562:111-116

73. Forsythe ID, Lambert DG, Nahorski SR, Linsdell P (1992) Elevation of cytosolic calcium by cholinoceptor agonists in SH-SY5Y human neuroblastoma cells: estimation of the contribution of voltage-dependent currents. Br J Pharmacol 107:207-214

74. Jalonen T, Akerman KEO (1988) Single transient potassium channels in human neuroblastoma cells induced to differentiate in vitro. Neurosci Lett 86:99-104

75. Reuveny E, Narahashi T (1993) Two types of high voltage-activated calcium channels in SH-SY5Y human neuroblastoma cells. Brain Res 603:64-73

76. Leventhal PS, Shelden EA, Kim B, Feldman EL (1997) Tyrosine phosphorylation of paxillin and focal adhesion kinase during insulin-like growth factor-I-stimulated lamellipodial advance. J Biol Chem 272:5214-5218

77. Leventhal PS, Feldman EL (1996) Tyrosine phosphorylation and enhanced expression of paxillin during neuronal differentiation in vitro. J Biol Chem 271:5957-5960

78. Leventhal PS, Feldman EL (1996) The tyrosine kinase inhibitor methyl 2,5-dihydroxycinnimate disrupts changes in the actin cytoskeleton required for neurite formation. Mol Brain Res 43:338-340

79. Recio-Pinto E, Ishii DN (1984) Effects of insulin, insulin-like growth factor-II and nerve growth factor on neurite outgrowth in cultured human neuroblastoma cells. Brain Res 302:323-334

80. Fernyhough P, Mill JF, Roberts JL, Ishii DN (1989) Stabilization of tubulin mRNAs by insulin and insulin-like growth factor I during neurite formation. Mol Brain Res 6:109-120

81. Recio-Pinto E, Ishii DN (1988) Insulin and insulin-like growth factor receptors regulating neurite formation in cultured human neuroblastoma cells. J Neurosci Res 19:312-320

82. Ishii DN, Wang C, Li Y (1991) Second messengers mediating gene expression essential to neurite formation directed by insulin and insulin-like growth factors. Adv Exp Med Biol 293:361-378

83. Kim B, Leventhal PS, Saltiel AR, Feldman EL (1997) Insulin-like growth factor (IGF)-I-mediated neurite outgrowth in vitro requires MAP kinase activation. J Biol Chem (in press)

84. Martin DM, Carlson RO, Feldman EL (1993) Interferon-g inhibits DNA synthesis and insulin-like growth factor-II expression in human neuroblastoma cells. J Neurosci Res 34:489-501

85. Sullivan KA, Kim B, Buzdon M, Feldman EL (1997) Suramin disrupts insulin-like growth factor-II (IGF-II) mediated autocrine growth in human SH-SY5Y neuroblastoma cells. Brain Res 744:199-206

86. Mattson ME, Hammerling U, Mohall E, Hall K, Pahlman S (1990) Mitogenically uncoupled insulin and IGF-I receptors of differentiated human neuroblastoma cells are functional and mediate ligand-induced signals. Growth Factors 2:251-265

87. Pahlman S, Meyerson G, Lindgren E, Schalling M, Johansson I (1991) Insulin-like growth factor I shifts from promoting cell division to potentiating maturation during neuronal differentiation. Proc Natl Acad Sci USA 88:9994-9998

88. Pahlman S, Mamaeva S, Meyerson G, Mattsson ME, Bjelfman C, Ortoft E, Hammerling U (1990) Human neuroblastoma cells in culture: a model for neuronal cell differentiation and function. Acta Physiol Scand Suppl 592:25-37

89. Thompson CB (1995) Apoptosis in the pathogenesis and treatment of disease. Science 267:1456-1462

90. Pittman RN, Wang S, Di Benedetto AJ, Mills JC (1993) A system for characterizing cellular and molecular events in programmed neuronal cell death. J Neurosci 13:3669-3680

91. Eastman A, Grant S, Lock R, Tritton T, Van Houten N, Yuan J (1994) Cell death in cancer and development: AACR special conference in cancer research. Cancer Res 54:2812-2818

92. Enokido Y, Akaneya Y, Niinobe M, Mikoshiba K, Hatanaka H (1992) Basic fibroblast growth factor rescues CNS neurons from cell death caused by high oxygen atmosphere in culture. Brain Res 599:261-271

93. D'Mello SR, Galli C, Ciotti T, Calissano P (1993) Induction of apoptosis in cerebellar granule neurons by low potassium: Inhibition of death by insulin-like growth factor I and cAMP. Proc Natl Acad Sci USA 90:10989-10993

94. Rukenstein A, Rydel RE, Greene LA (1991) Multiple agents resue PC12 cells from serum-free cell death by translation- and transcription-independent mechanisms. J Neurosci 11:2552-2563

95. Raff MC, Barres BA, Burne JF, Coles HS, Ishizaki Y, Jacobson MD (1994) Programmed cell death and the control of cell survival: Lessons from the nervous system. Science 262:695-700

96. Stewart BW (1994) Mechanisms of apoptosis: integration of genetic, biochemical, and cellular indicators. J Natl Cancer Inst 86:1286-1296

97. Reed JC (1994) Bcl-2 and the regulation of programmed cell death. J Cell Biol 124:1-6

98. Jacobson MD, Evan GI (1994) Breaking the ice. Structural and functional similarities have been discovered between two mammalian proteins, Bcl-2 and interleukin 1b-converting enzyme, and proteins encoded by nematode cell-death genes. Curr Biol 4:337-340

99. Baur AM, Gamberger TI, Weerda HG, Gjuric M, Tamm ER (1995) Laminin promotes differentiation, adhesion and proliferation of cell cultures derived from human acoustic nerve schwannoma. Acta Otolaryngol (Stockh) 115:517-521

100. Hockenbery D, Nunez G, Milliman C, Schreiber RD, Korsmeyer SJ (1990) Bcl-2 is an inner mitochondrial membrane protein that blocks programmed cell death. Nature 348:334-336

101. Bissonette RP, Echeverri F, Mahboubi A, Green DR (1992) Apoptotic cell death induced by c-myc is inhibited by Bcl-2. Nature 359:552-554

102. Merry DE, Veis DJ, Hickey WF, Korsmeyer SJ (1994) Bcl-2 protein expression is widespread in the developing nervous system and retained in the adult PNS. Development 120:301-311

103. Boise LH, Gonzalez-Garcia M, Postema CE, Ding L, Lindsten T, Turka LA, Mao X, Nunez G, Thompson CB (1993) Bcl-x, a Bcl-2-related gene that functions as a dominant regulator of apoptotic cell death. Cell 74:597-608

104. Martinou J-C, Dubois-Dauphin M, Staple JK, Rodriguez I, Frankowski H, Missotten M, Albertini P, Talabot D, Catsicas S, Pietra C, Huarte J (1994) Overexpression of Bcl-2 in transgenic mice protects neurons from naturally occurring cell death and experimental ischemia. Neuron 13:1017-1030

105. Allsopp TE, Wyatt S, Paterson HF, Davies AM (1994) The proto-oncogene Bcl-2 can selectively rescue neurotrophic factor-dependent neurons from apoptosis. Cell 73:295-307

106. Garcia I, Martinou I, Tsujimoto Y, Martinou J-C (1992) Prevention of programmed cell death of sympathetic neurons by the Bcl-2 proto-oncogene. Science 258:302-304

107. Mah SP, Zhong LT, Liu Y, Roghani A, Edwards RH, Bredesen DE (1993) The protooncogene Bcl-2 inhibits apoptosis in PC12 cells. J Neurochem 60:1183-1186

108. Roth KA, Motoyama N, Loh DY (1996) Apoptosis of Bcl-x-deficient telencephalic cells in vitro. J Neurosci 16:1753-1758

109. Tewari M, Dixit VM (1995) Fas-and tumor necrosis factor-induced apoptosis is inhibited by the poxvirus crmA gene product. J Biol Chem 270:3255-3260

110. Chinnaiyan AM, O'Rourke K, Tewari M, Dixit VM (1995) FADD, a novel death domain-containing protein, interacts with the death domain of Fas and initiates apoptosis. Cell 81:505-512

111. Tewari M, Beidler DR, Dixit VM (1995) CrmA-inhibitable cleavage of the 70-kDa protein component of the U1 small nuclear ribonucleoprotein during fas- and tumor necrosis factor-induced apoptosis. J Biol Chem 270:18738-18741

112. Tewari M, Quan LT, O'Rourke K, Desnoyers S, Zheng Z, Beidler DR, Poirier GG, Salvesen GS, Dixit VM (1995) Yama/CPP32b, a mammalian homolog of CED-3, is a CrmA-inhibitable protease that cleaves the death substrate poly(ADP-ribose) polymerase. Cell 81:801-809

113. Schlegel J, Peters I, Orrenius S, Miller DK, Thornberry NA, Yamin T-T, Nicholson DW (1996) CPP32/apopain is a key interleukin 1b converting enzyme-like protease involved in fas-mediated apoptosis. J Biol Chem 271:1841-1844

114. Darmon AJ, Nicholson DW, Bleackley RC (1995) Activation of the apoptotic protease CPP32 by cytotoxic T-cell-derived granzyme B. Nature 377:446-448

115. Duan H, Chinnaiyan AM, Hudson PL, Wing JP, He W-W, Dixit VM (1996) ICE-LAP3, a novel mammalian homologue of the Caenorhabditis elegans cell death protein Ced-3 is activated during Fas- and tumor necrosis factor-induced apoptosis. J Biol Chem 271:1621-1625

116. Chinnaiyan AM, Dixit VM (1996) The cell death machine. Curr Biol 6:555-562

117. Chinnaiyan AM, Orth K, O'Rourke K, Duan H, Poirer GG, Dixit VM (1996) Molecular

ordering of the cell death pathway: Bcl-2 and Bcl-X$_L$ function upstream of the CED-3-like apoptotic proteases. J Biol Chem 271:4573-4576

118. Kaufmann SH, Desnoyers S, Ottaviano Y, Davidson NE, Poirier GG (1993) Specific proteolytic cleavage of poly(ADP-ribose) polymerase: An early marker of chemotherapy-induced apoptosis. Cancer Res 53:3976-3985

119. Corkins MR, Vanderhoof JA, Slentz DH, MacDonald RG, Park JHY (1995) Growth stimulation by transfection of intestinal epithelial cells with an antisense insulin-like growth factor binding protein-2 construct. Biochem Biophys Res Commun 211:707-713

120. Korsmeyer SJ (1995) Regulators of cell death. Trends Genet 11:101-105

121. Corcoran GB, Fix L, Jones DP, Moslen MT, Nicotera P, Oberhammer FA, Buttyan R (1994) Contemporary issues in toxicology. Apoptosis: molecular control point in toxicity. Toxicol Appl Pharmacol 128:169-181

122. Wyllie AH (1995) The genetic regulation of apoptosis. Curr Opin Genet Dev 5:97-104

123. Matthews CC, Feldman EL (1996) Insulin-like growth factor I rescues SH-SY5Y human neuroblastoma cells from hyperosmotic induced programmed cell death. J Cell Physiol 166:323-331

124. Singleton JR, Randolph AE, Feldman EL (1996) Insulin-like growth factor I receptor prevents apotosis and enhances neuroblastoma tumorigenesis. Cancer Res 56:4522-4529

125. Singleton JR, Dixit VM, Feldman EL (1996) Type I insulin-like growth factor receptor activation regulates apoptotic proteins. J Biol Chem 271:31791-31794

126. Matthews C, Odeh H, Feldman EL (1996) Insulin-like growth factor-I is an osmoprotectant in human neuroblastoma cells. Neuroscience (in press)

127. Muta K, Krantz SB, Bondurant MC, Wickrema A (1994) Distinct roles of erythropoietin, insulin-like growth factor I, and stem cell factor in the development of erythroid progenitor cells. J Clin Invest 94:34-43

128. Shapiro DN, Jones BG, Shapiro LH, Dias P, Houghton PJ (1994) Antisense-mediated reduction in insulin-like growth factor-I receptor expression suppresses the malignant phenotype of a human alveolar rhabdomyosarcoma. J Clin Invest 94:1235-1242

129. Trojan J, Blossey BK, Johnson TR, Rudin SD, Tykocinski M, Ilan J (1992) Loss of tumorigenicity of rat glioblastoma directed by episome-based antisense cDNA transcription of insulin-like growth factor I. Proc Natl Acad Sci USA 89:4874-4878

130. Resnicoff M, Sell C, Rubini M, Coppola D, Ambrose D, Baserga R, Rubin R (1994) Rat glioblastoma cells expressing an antisense RNA to the insulin-like growth factor-1 (IGF-1) receptor are nontumorigenic and induce regression of wild-type tumors. Cancer Res 54:2218-2222

131. Resnicoff M, Coppola D, Sell C, Rubin R, Ferrone S, Baserga R (1994) Growth inhibition of human melanoma cells in nude mice by antisense strategies to the type 1 insulin-like growth factor receptor. Cancer Res 54:4848-4850

132. Yao R, Cooper GM (1995) Requirement for phosphatidylinositol-3 kinase in the prevention of apoptosis by nerve growth factor. Science 267:2003-2006

Insulin-like Growth Factor I: Regulation and Interactions During Aging-Induced Cognitive Decline and Impairment Within the Hippocampus

P. K. Lund[1], K. L. Stenvers[2], M. Gallagher[3]

Introduction

A considerable body of evidence indicates that hippocampal circuitry is especially vulnerable to the neurodegeneration associated with normal and pathological aging. However, aged hippocampus appears to retain some of its capacity to regenerate in response to this damage [1-3]. Axonal sprouting and synaptic reorganization have been reported in hippocampal regions sustaining loss of cells or input during normal aging [2, 3]. Neurotrophic factors (NTFs) are believed to be necessary for such structural reorganization. One family of NTFs, the insulin-like growth factors (IGFs), may have actions on a broad spectrum of hippocampal cells [4-10]. This family of growth factors consists of two peptides, IGF-I and IGF-II, which interact with two different receptors, the type 1 and type 2 IGF receptors (IGFR). The type 1 IGFR, which has high affinity for both IGFs, mediates many of the proliferative and differentiative actions of the IGFs [9, 10]. The functional role of the type 2 receptor, which has high affinity for IGF-II but low affinity for IGF-I, is not well defined [11-14]. The IGF system also includes a family of six IGF binding proteins (IGFBPs) that modulate IGF action and availability in tissue-, cell-, and development-specific manners [9, 10].

Extensive research has demonstrated the neurotrophic actions of IGFs during central nervous system (CNS) development, in which they promote the growth, survival, and differentiation of neurons and glia [9, 10]. Studies in mature brain suggest that IGFs continue to provide the neurotrophic support necessary for neuronal repair and survival in adult rat brain. In the adult rat hippocampal formation, in situ hybridization histochemistry has established the presence of transcripts for IGF-I [11], the type 1 and type 2 IGFRs [6, 11], and at least one IGF binding protein, IGFBP-4 [8, 12]. In vitro autoradiographic receptor binding assays have demonstrated high ^{125}I-IGF-I binding in the neuropil layers of the hippocampus in the vicinity of cells producing IGF-I messenger RNA (mRNA) [7]. Recent evidence suggests that the IGFs can cross the blood-brain barrier [13]. Thus, IGF-I may influence hippocampal function in

[1]Department of Physiology and Curriculum in Neurobiology, University of North Carolina, Chapel Hill, North Carolina, USA, [2]Ludwig Institute for Cancer Research, Melbourne, Australia and [3]Department of Psychology, Johns Hopkins University, Baltimore, Maryland, USA

endocrine, paracrine, and autocrine fashions via interactions with the type 1 receptor. The actions of IGF-I in adult brain may be modulated by IGFBP-4. Several components of the IGF system are regulated in response to damage in the hippocampal formation or in its afferent cell populations [7, 10, 14-18], suggesting that IGFs are involved in neuronal survival and repair processes. Since structural damage and loss of input can occur in normally aged hippocampus, IGFs may also be involved in regenerative or maintenance processes in aged brain. IGF-I and IGF-II mRNAs are present in aged rat brain but at reduced levels compared to young adult brain [17, 18]. Little or no information is available about the levels of expression of IGFs, IGF receptors, and IGFBPs in different regions of aged brain or about their regulation during cognitive decline. In order to establish if the hippocampal IGF system plays a role in aging-induced decline in cognitive function we have asked a number of questions as follows:

Do the Sites of Expression of IGF-I, Type I IGFR and IGFBP-4 Change in Aged Compared with Young Adult Hippocampus?

In situ hybridization histochemistry was used to compare the distribution patterns of IGF-I, type 1 IGFR and IGFBPs in young adult and aged hippocampus. Of the six IGFBPs, only IGFBP-4 is expressed at high levels in the hippocampus of adult rat [8]. Particularly high IGFBP-4 expression was found in pyramidal neurons of the subfields of Ammon's horn and the subiculum, and in the granule cell layer of the anterior hippocampal continuation (Table 1). In situ hybridiza-

Table 1. Distribution of IGFBP-4 and IGFBP5 mRNAs in adult rat forebrain

Brain region		IGFBP-4 mRNA	IGFBP-5 mRNA
Olfactory system	Olfactory bulb, periglomerular cells	-	++
	Anterior olfactory nucleus	+++	-
	Ventral tenia tecta	++	-
	Amygdaloid complex	+	-
Striatel area	Caudate-putamen	+	-
	Nucleus accumbens	+	-
Hippocampal formation	Dorsal tenia tecta, granule cell layer	++++	-
	Indusium griseum, granule cell layer	++++	-
	Dorsal CA1, pyramidal cell layer	++++	-
	Dorsal CA2, pyramidal cell layer	++	-
	Anterior CA3, pyramidal cell layer	+++	-
	Ventral hippocampus, CA subfields	+	-
	Dentate gyrus, polymorphic zone	+	-
	Subiculum, pyramidal cell layer	++++	-
	Parasubiculum	+	-
	Presubiculum	++	-

Expression levels: -, undetectable; +, low; ++, moderate; +++, high; ++++, intense

tion histochemistry revealed no qualitative differences between the distribution patterns for IGFBP-4 mRNAs in young adult and aged hippocampus [8, 18]. The distribution patterns of type 1 IGFR and IGF-I mRNAs in aged rat brain corresponded to those previously reported in young adult rat brain [1, 5, 18]. Type 1 receptor mRNA was highly abundant in the granule cell layer of the dentate gyrus and in the pyramidal cell layer of the entire CA3 subfield (Fig. 1). Lesser levels of expression were evident in other CA subfields and in the polymorphic zone of the dentate gyrus. IGF-I mRNA expression was restricted to isolated cells of the neuropil layers of the CA subfields and dentate gyrus of the hippocampal formation (data not shown). No difference was observed between the distribution patterns of IGF-I mRNA in young and aged brain [18].

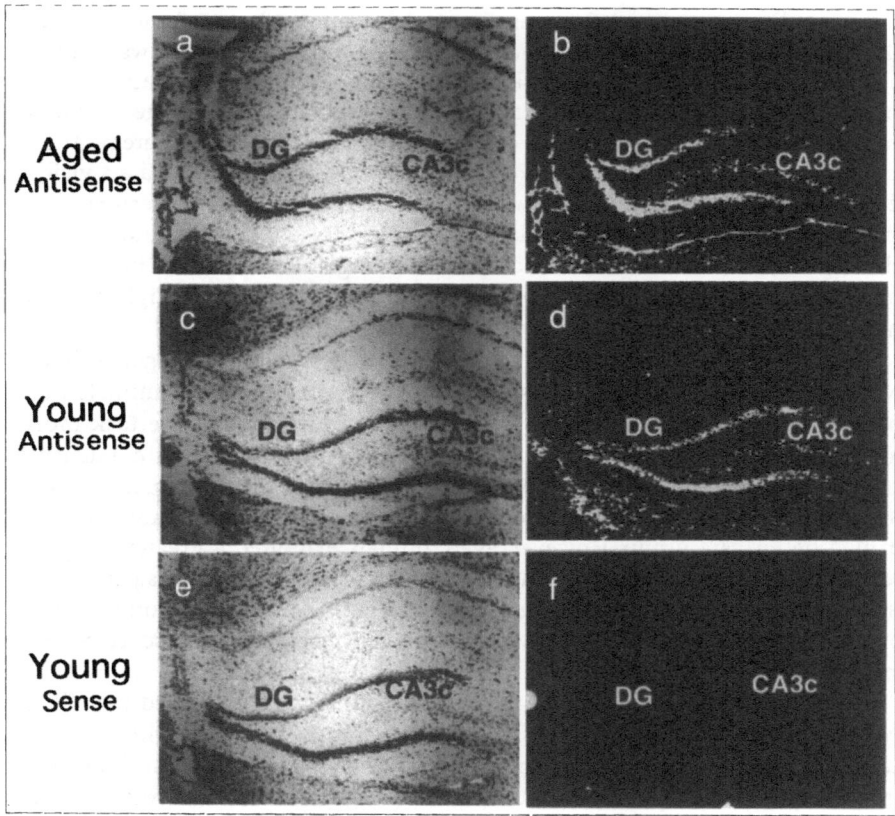

Fig. 1a-f. Type 1 IGF receptor mRNA in the dorsal hippocampal formation of aged and young rats visualized by in situ hybridization histochemistry. Paired light-field (**a, c, e**) and dark-field (**b, d, f**) low-power photomicrographs. The type 1 receptor antisense cRNA probe showed similar hybridization patterns in sections of aged (**b**) and young (**d**) dentate gyrus (*DG*). Hybridization was particularly heavy in the granule cell layer of the dentate gyrus and in the pyramidal cell layer of the CA3 subfield of the hippocampus (only CA3c visible). **e, f** Type 1 receptor sense RNA probe showed no hybridization in a section adjacent to that in **d**. *CA3c* = CA subfield of the hippocampal formation

Do Changes in the Levels of IGF Gene Expression Correlate with Age or Cognitive Impairment?

During aging, functional deterioration of a particular system such as the hippocampus occurs in only a subset of animals, indicating that there are individual differences in susceptibility to aging-induced impairment. Comparisons between young adult and aged animals may not reveal or may under-represent those aging-induced changes associated with functional impairment [19]. It is with this in mind that our studies include behavioral testing of young and aged animals for cognitive function. Spatial learning impairment in rodents, a model of cognitive decline, likely reflects neurobiological aging in forebrain systems including hippocampus and forebrain projections to the hippocampus [19, 20]. In our studies, spatial learning was assessed in young adult (7-8 months) and aged (28-29 months) male, pathogen-free Long-Evans rats using a water maze task [18-20]. Briefly, rats were trained to locate a submerged platform in a water-filled, circular tank. Probe trials were interpolated during the course of training to assess the development of a spatially guided learning strategy. At the completion of this testing, rats were assessed for their ability to locate a visible platform without spatial guides within the maze environment. Performance accuracy was assessed using cumulative search errors and learning index scores which provide measures of distance from the target. Lower scores indicated a more accurate search in the vicinity of the target location while higher scores indicated a more random search and poor spatial learning ability.

Figure 2 shows mean cumulative search error for young and aged animals over four blocks of training trials. Initially, the young and aged animals performed similarly, but the young animals as a group learned the task more quickly than did the aged group, as indicated by the lower mean cumulative search error on repeated trials (Fig. 2a). Comparisons of individual learning index scores for the young and aged animals revealed that young animals performed better as a group. However, aged animals exhibited a greater range of performances than did the young animals, and some of the aged rats performed as well as the young adult rats (Fig. 2b). Only a subset of the aged animals performed outside the range of the young animals (learning index score > 250) and were considered severely impaired on the spatial task (Fig. 2b).

Hippocampi from the behaviorally tested animals were assayed for IGF-I, type 1 IGFR and IGFBP-4 mRNA abundance using northern hybridization or ribonuclease protection (RNase protection) assays. An important feature of aging is that the changes which occur are often smaller than those which occur in disease or in disease models such as brain lesions [22-24]. Therefore, quantitative assays must be sufficiently sensitive and precise to detect relatively small changes. With this in mind, RNA extractions and analyses were performed simultaneously on all hippocampus specimens from the study group to minimize inter-assay variation and to maximize detection of small differences in mRNA abundance. Assays have been described in detail [18]. Table 2 shows the mean abundance of type 1 IGFR, IGF-I and IGFBP-4 mRNAs in young and aged

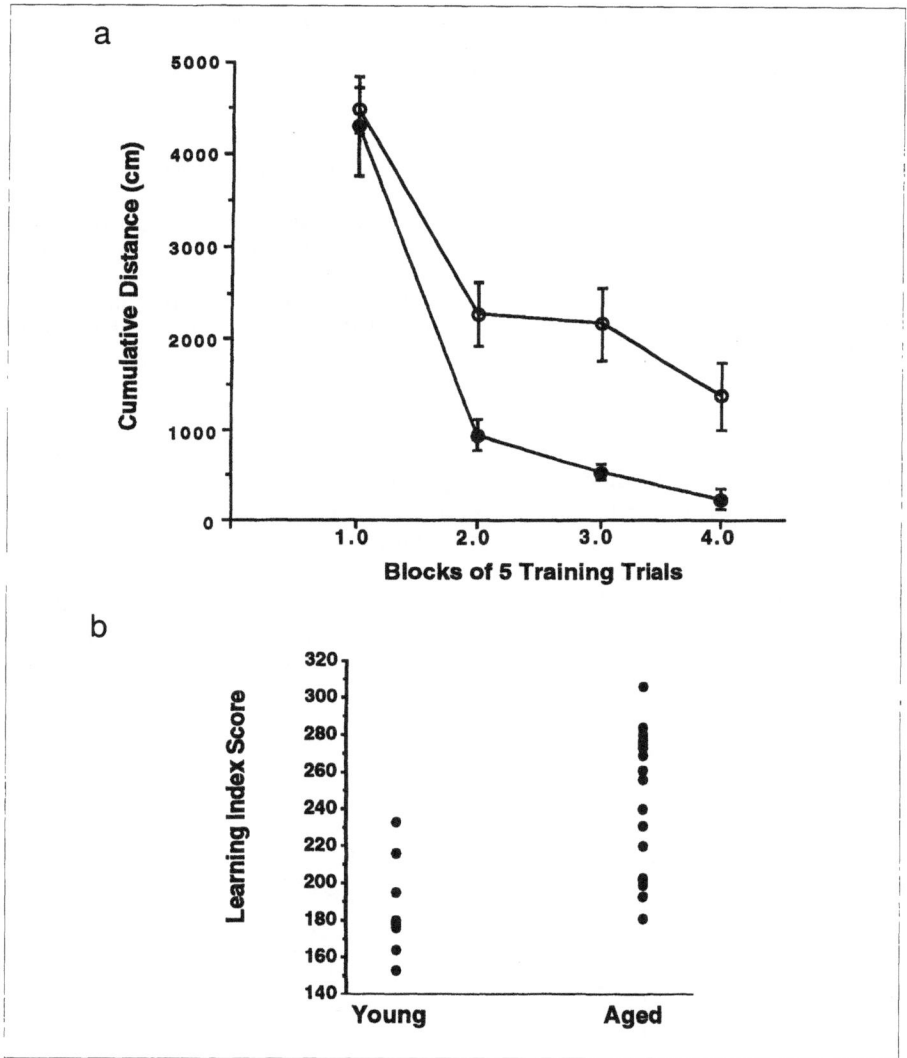

Fig. 2a, b. Age-related behavioral impairment in the Morris water maze. **a** Differences in performance between the young (*filled circles*) and aged (*open circles*) groups over the course of training on the spatial version of the water maze. Cumulative distance (±SEM), averaged across blocks of five training trials, is a reflection of the proximity of the animal to the target throughout the trial. **b** Distribution of the individual learning index scores calculated from probe trials for the young and aged rats used in the quantitative assays of IGF mRNAs

hippocampus. Statistical analysis revealed a significant age-related increase in the type 1 IGFR mRNA within the hippocampal formation of aged rats ($t = 2.50$, $P < 0.02$). In contrast, there was no significant difference between young and aged hippocampi for either IGF-I or IGFBP-4 mRNA abundance. Linear

Table 2. Abundance of IGF mRNAs in young- and aged-rat hippocampus

	Type 1 IGFR	IGF-I	IGFBP-4
Young	0.179 ± 0.01 (n = 8)	0.123 ± 0.02 (n = 5)	0.565 ± 0.10 (n = 5)
Aged	0.218 ± 0.01* (n = 17)	0.115 ± 0.01 (n = 13)	0.499 ± 0.04 (n = 15)

mRNA abundance is expressed in arbitrary units as mean ± SEM; values are derived from the ratio of the optical density of the specific mRNA signal to that of the respective control mRNAs

n = number of test subjects for each assay. n is not constant because limiting amounts of total RNA extracted from individual hippocampi precluded assay of all three mRNAs in a subset of samples

*$P < 0.02$ for young vs. aged

regression indicated that type 1 receptor mRNA expression was significantly correlated with learning index scores (Fig. 3). Neither IGF-I ($r = 0.17$, $P = -0.50$; n = 18) nor IGFBP-4 ($r = 0.01$, $P = 0.98$; n = 20) mRNA abundance was significantly related to the learning index scores. Linear regression revealed a significant correlation between IGF-I and type 1 receptor mRNA abundance, such that lower IGF-I mRNA abundance was associated with higher type 1 receptor mRNA expression ($r = -0.72$, $P < 0.01$; n = 13). This relationship followed a similar trend across all subjects but did not reach statistical significance overall

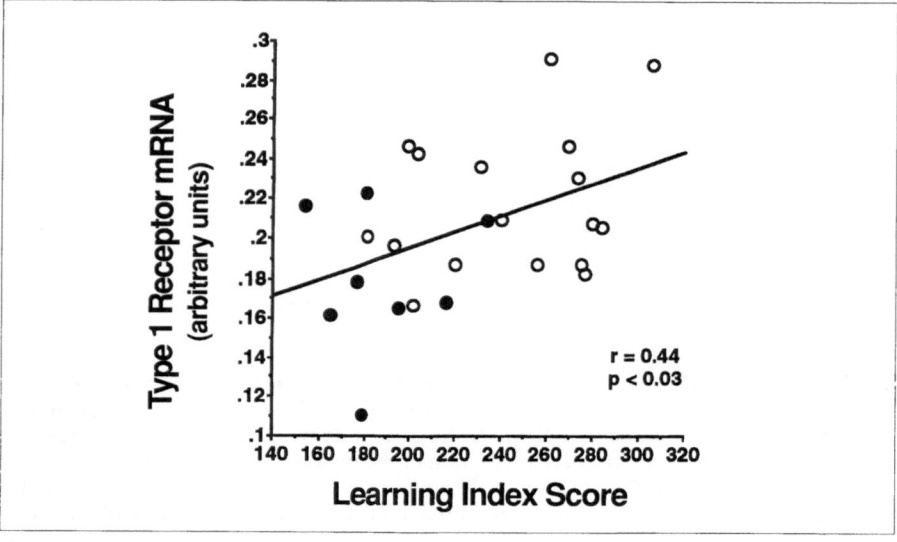

Fig. 3. Relationship between learning index scores and the abundance of type 1 receptor mRNAs in total RNA extracted from individual young (*filled circles*) and aged (*open circles*) rat hippocampi. Note that lower values for the learning index scores represent better spatial learning. The line was determined by linear regression analysis. Pearson's correlation coefficient and significance are given

($r = -0.46$, $P < 0.06$; n = 18). No significant relationships were revealed between the abundance of IGFBP-4 mRNA and either IGF-I or type 1 receptor mRNA.

The age-related increase in type 1 receptor mRNA could reflect a number of underlying regulatory events. The negative correlation between abundance of IGF-I and type 1 receptor mRNAs in the hippocampi of individual rats suggests that IGF-I availability may have some impact on receptor expression in brain, especially in aged rats. Levels of type 1 receptor mRNA expression and IGF binding show a similar reciprocal relationship with levels of IGF peptide in several peripheral tissues [21]. Other sources of IGFs may be available to the hippocampus and may regulate type 1 receptor mRNA expression. IGFs can cross the blood-brain barrier by receptor-mediated transport [14]. The extent to which the IGFs cross into the hippocampus appears to be low in normal adult rat, and it is currently unclear whether the peripheral circulation represents a significant source of IGF peptide for the hippocampal formation. Levels of circulating IGF-I are reduced with age in humans and rats [21, 22], indicating a potential loss of trophic endocrine support available to the CNS.

A reduction in IGF-II, which binds the type 1 receptor with high affinity, could also contribute to the regulation of type 1 receptor mRNA in the hippocampus. Although IGF-II mRNA is not locally synthesized in the hippocampus, IGF-II may access the hippocampus by way of the cerebrospinal fluid (CSF), where it is found at high levels in adults [23]. IGF-II mRNA is decreased in aged rat brain compared to young rat brain [21, 22], presumably reflecting a decrease in IGF-II expression within the leptomeninges and choroid plexus where high levels of IGF-II transcripts have been detected by in situ hybridization [7, 10].

A decrease in IGF availability by any of the above mechanisms could leave hippocampal cells susceptible to degenerative processes and contribute to the up-regulation of type 1 receptor mRNA. In view of the lack of direct evidence for an age-related decrease in IGF availability within the hippocampal formation, alternative hypotheses must be considered to account for the increase in type 1 IGF receptor mRNA with age. One possible explanation is that the increase in expression may occur in response to degenerative or regenerative processes that occur within the hippocampal formation with age. Such processes have been well documented in normally and pathologically aged brain [29, 30]. With this in mind we undertook studies to assess if deafferentation of inputs to the hippocampus alters expression of the IGF system within the hippocampus.

Do Lesions that Mimic Aging-Induced Deafferentation of the Hippocampus Alter Expression of the IGF System?

Partial deafferentation of the hippocampus occurs during normal aging and, to a more severe degree, in Alzheimer's disease [19, 24]. Within the dentate gyrus, roughly a third of the synapses from the entorhinal perforant pathway are lost in normal aged brain. A second major afferent projection to the hippocampus, the cholinergic basal forebrain projection, also undergoes atrophy during normal and pathological aging. A number of regenerative events in the hippocampus accompany this degeneration, including axonal sprouting, dendritic reorganization, and glial proliferation [1, 3, 25]. Studies in which one or both of these pathways are lesioned in young adult rats have reproduced some of the neurobiological aspects of hippocampal aging. For example, entorhinal cortex lesions remove perforant path input to the outer molecular layer of the dentate gyrus, and result in a well-characterized sprouting response of septal afferents and commissural and associational fibers into the deafferented area [25]. Fimbria-fornix transections, which remove non-cholinergic as well as cholinergic basal forebrain projections to the hippocampal formation, similarly induce sprouting of surviving afferents within hippocampal terminal fields [25, 26]. The patterns of sprouting induced by these experimental lesions of hippocampal afferents resemble that observed in normally aged rat brain.

Preliminary studies were performed in young adult animals with either of two lesions that mimicked different aspects of hippocampus deafferentation associated with aging. In one set of animals, the entorhinal cortex was bilaterally aspirated to mimic loss of perforant pathway input to the dentate gyrus observed with age. IGF mRNAs were quantified in hippocampi of lesioned animals and sham-operated controls ($t = 3.05$; $P < 0.01$) 14 days after treatment. These studies revealed that entorhinal lesion is associated with a significant increase in hippocampal IGF-I mRNA abundance when compared to sham-lesioned controls [27]. This is in agreement with recent reports of increased IGF-I expression within the deafferented areas of the hippocampus and dentate gyrus following unilateral entorhinal lesions [7, 15]. There is no significant effect of bilateral entorhinal lesion on abundance of either type 1 receptor or IGFBP-4 mRNA within the hippocampus [27]. Thus entorhinal lesions in young rats did not mimic our previously observed changes in the IGF system with aging in that there is no compensatory increase in expression of type 1 receptor as observed with aging. In contrast to aging, entorhinal lesion induced an increase in hippocampal IGF-I mRNA which may reflect a response to the extensive tissue damage from the lesion. Many situations of CNS damage are known to be associated with increased local IGF-I expression [10, 14].

In a separate set of animals, 192 IgG saporin was bilaterally injected into the medial septum (MS) and vertical limb of the diagonal band (VDB) of Broca (Fig. 4). 192 IgG saporin is an immunotoxin comprising a ribosome-inactivating cytotoxin coupled to a monoclonal antibody against the low-affinity p75 neurotrophin receptor [28]. Intraparenchymal injection of 192 IgG saporin into the MS/VDB area has been shown to deplete a number of cholinergic markers in the basal forebrain and hippocampal terminal fields, while largely sparing non-cholinergic neurons in the basal forebrain [28]. Thus, use of this immunotoxin allows for the selective removal of the cholinergic basal forebrain projection to the hippocampal formation. Animals were studied at 14 days after injection of the immunotoxin or vehicle. Assays of choline-acetyltransferase (ChAT) within the hippocampus revealed a decrease in the lesioned animals confirming

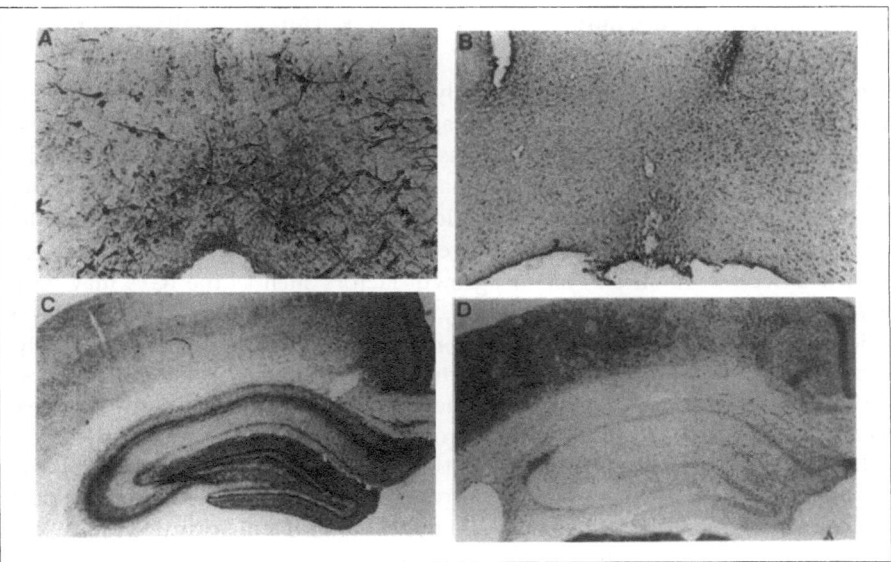

Fig. 4a-d. ChAT immunochemistry in the medial septal/vertical diagonal band region (MS/VBD) and acetylcholinesterase (AChE) staining in dorsal hippocampus. **a** Lower portion of the MS/VBD region in a control brain that contained neurons immunoreactive for anti-ChAT antibody. **b** Absence of ChAT-positive neurons in an experimental brain (MS/VBD) injected with the immunotoxin 192 IgG saporin. **c** AChE staining in control hippocampus. **d** AChE staining in MS/VDB-lesioned hippocampus. x40

the efficacy of the lesion [27]. Immunotoxin-mediated lesion of cholinergic input to the hippocampus resulted in a significant increase in hippocampal type 1 receptor mRNA in lesioned rats compared to rats that received vehicle injections at surgery ($t = 2.56$; $P < 0.02$), but no significant effect on either IGF-I or IGFBP-4 mRNA abundance [27]. In intact adult rat brain, type 1 receptor mRNA is abundant in the pyramidal neurons of the CA subfields and granule cells of the dentate gyrus, and IGF-I binding is localized in the adjacent neuropil layers [5, 7]. Since cholinergic basal forebrain afferents terminate on dendrites throughout these areas [29], removal of cholinergic afferents denervates neurons expressing type 1 receptor mRNA. Thus, type 1 receptor up-regulation within hippocampal neurons may support dendritic retraction and regrowth in response to the loss of afferents and promote subsequent ingrowth of new fibers. The effect of the cholinergic basal forebrain lesion to increase hippocampal type 1 IGF receptor mRNA resembles the effect of aging on hippocampal type 1 IGF receptor expression, suggesting that the loss of cholinergic input to the hippocampus contributes to the age-related alterations in type 1 IGF receptor gene expression. This hypothesis is amenable to future testing using pharmacological approaches.

What is the Functional Role of the IGF System Within Aging Hippocampus?

The studies described above provide only a descriptive starting point to understanding the functional role of IGFs in aged hippocampus. Altered IGF expression could be a causative factor in loss of cognitive function. Alternatively, altered expression of the IGF system may be an epiphenomenon secondary to neurobiological and cognitive dysfunction. It is clearly desirable to define the functional role of the IGF system in aged hippocampus and in aging-induced cognitive decline. As in all systems, growth factors such as the IGFs may have dual functional identities. During aging, optimal growth factor expression and action may be required for optimal neuronal survival and function. Alternatively, local increases in growth factor or growth factor receptor expression may represent a tissue response to localized damage and could contribute to cognitive decline by inducing aberrant, reactive growth. Systemic or local administration of the IGFs to aged animals in conjunction with behavioral testing represents one approach to testing the functional role of the IGFs in the neurobiological and cognitive changes that occur with aging. One problem with this approach, which is a general problem in the aging field, is that the timing and duration of growth factor treatment may be critical in terms of cognitive effects and it may be difficult to alter IGF status over the time-frame required to alter cognitive function.

Transgenic models offer the potential for long-term manipulation of growth factor status that may be required to fully define their role in aging. An increasing number of transgenic models with specific alterations in the IGF system are available [10]. Altered brain size, myelination and numbers of hippocampal neurons in models of IGF-I excess [10], IGF-I deficiency [4, 10] or altered IGF-I action [10] point to an important role of IGF-I in hippocampal function. Behavioral testing of these mouse models during aging could provide insights into the long-term functional effects of IGF-I within the hippocampus and in cognitive function. The application of behavioral testing to transgenic and gene knockout mice is a new but exciting direction.

Interactions of IGF-I with Other Hormones and Growth Factors

A hallmark of IGF-I action is that its individual mitogenic, survival or differentiative effects are often weak but it modulates the actions of other hormones and growth factors [30]. Interactions between growth hormone (GH) and IGF-I in regulating somatic growth are well established. Excess IGF-I can compensate for the reduced brain size observed in GH-deficient transgenic mice [10]. Little is known about the behavioral consequences of perturbations in GH and IGF-I expression. Behavioral testing of the transgenic mice used to assess relative effects of GH and IGF-I on somatic growth and organ size could provide useful insights into these hormones' effects on cognitive function. This is an interesting and important issue as recombinant GH and IGF-I are used increasingly in the clinical setting and, in some situations, in aged individuals.

In several model cell systems such as fibroblasts and keratinocytes, it is clear that progression through the cell cycle requires IGF-I in combination with another growth factor acting through a receptor tyrosine kinase (e.g. platelet-derived growth factor (PDGF) or epidermal growth factor (EGF)) [31]. One recent study demonstrated synergistic mitogenic effects of EGF and IGF-I associated with effects of EGF on the expression of type 1 IGF receptor and IGFBPs but differential effects of EGF and IGF-I on intracellular signaling pathways leading to transcriptional activation of c-*fos* and c-*jun* [3]. Other studies found synergistic, anti-apoptotic activities of EGF and IGF-I [32]. IGF-I altered the responsiveness of some model neuronal systems to other growth factors such as NGF and to other hormones such as estrogen [10]. However, the interactions between IGF-I and other growth factors and hormones within the nervous system remain largely unexplored and represent a fruitful and important future direction.

IGF-I and IGF-II are induced at sites of tissue damage, including damage within the nervous system [10, 14, 33]. The mediators of IGF induction in response to damage of the nervous system are not defined, but evidence from other systems points to a role of pro-inflammatory cytokines [33]. Localized tissue injury in the brain or hippocampus may be associated with aging and may similarly induce IGF expression via cytokine-mediated mechanisms. Identifying and modulating such mechanisms will likely contribute to our understanding of the role of IGFs in aging-induced neurobiological and cognitive decline.

Acknowledgments

The authors' work is supported by NIH grant AG09973.

References

1. Hefti F (1994) Neurotrophic factor therapy for nervous system degenerative diseases. J Neurobiol 25:1418-1435
2. Flood DG, Coleman PD (1988) Neuron numbers and sizes in aging brain: comparison of human, monkey, and rodent brain. Neurobiol Aging 9:453-463
3. Flood DG, Coleman PD (1990) Hippocampal plasticity in normal aging and decreased plasticity in Alzheimer's disease. Prog Brain Res 83:453-443
4. Beck KD, Powell-Braxton L, Widmer H-R, Valverde J, Hefti F (1995) IGF1 gene disruption results in reduced brain size, CNS hypomyelination, and loss of hippocampal granule and striatal parvalbumin-containing neurons. Neuron 14:717-730
5. Bondy CA, Werner H, Roberts CT Jr, LeRoith D (1992) Cellular pattern of type 1 insulin-like growth factor receptor gene expression during maturation of the rat brain: Comparison with insulin-like growth factors I and II. Neuroscience 46:909-923
6. Couce ME, Weatherington AJ, McGinty JF (1992) Expression of insulin-like growth fac-

tor-II (IGF-II) and IGF-II/mannose-6-phosphate receptor in the rat hippocampus: an in situ hybridization and immunocytochemical study. Endocrinology 131:1636-1642

7.   Kar S, Baccichet A, Quirion R, Poirier J (1993) Entorhinal cortex lesion induces differential responses in [125I] insulin-like growth factor I, [125I] insulin-like growth factor II, and [125I] insulin receptor binding sites in the rat hippocampal formation. Neuroscience 55:69-80

8.   Stenvers KL, Zimmermann EM, Gallagher M, Lund PK (1994) Expression of insulin-like growth factor binding protein-4 and -5 mRNAs in adult rat forebrain. J Comp Neurol 339:91-105

9.   Hepler JE, Lund PK (1990) Molecular biology of the insulin-like growth factors: relevance to nervous system function. Mol Neurobiol 2:93-127

10. D'Ercole AJ, Ping Y, Calikoghi AS, Ospiana GG (1996) The role of the insulin-like growth factors in the central nervous system. Mol Neurobiol 13:227-255

11. Bondy C (1991) Transient IGF I gene expression during maturation of functionally related central projection neurons. J Neurosci 11:3442-3455

12. Brar AK, Chernausek SD (1993) Localization of insulin-like growth factor binding protein-4 expression in the developing and adult rat brain: analysis by in situ hybridization. J Neurosci Res 35:103-114

13. Reinhardt RR, Bondy CA (1994) Insulin-like growth factors cross the blood brain barrier. Endocrinology 135:1753-1761

14. Gluckman PD, Guan J, Beiharz EJ, Klempt ND, Klempt M, Miller O, Sirimanne E, Dragunow M, Williams CE (1993) The role of the insulin-like growth factor system in neuronal rescue. Ann N Y Acad Sci 692:138-148

15. Guthrie KM, Nguyen T, Gall CM (1995) Insulin-like growth factor-1 mRNA is increased in deafferented hippocampus: spatiotemporal correspondence of a trophic event with axon sprouting. J Comp Neurol 352:147-160

16. Kitraki E, Bozas E, Philippidis H, Stylianopoulou F (1993) Aging-related changes in IGF-II and c-fos gene expression in the rat brain. Int J Dev Neurosci 11:1-9

17. Park GH, Buetow DE (1991) Genes for insulin-like growth factors I and II are expressed in senescent rat tissues. Gerontology 37:310-316

18. Stenvers KL, Lund PK, Gallagher M (1996) Increased expression of type 1 insulin-like growth factor receptor messenger RNA in rat hippocampal formation is associated with aging and behavioral impairment. Neuroscience 72:505-518

19. Gallagher M, Gill TM, Baxter MG, Bucci DJ (1994) The development of neurobiological models for cognitive decline in aging. Semin Neurosci 6:351-358

20. Gallagher M, Burwell R, Burchinal M (1993) Severity of spatial learning impairment in aging: development of a learning index score for performance in the Morris water maze. Behav Neurosci 107:618-626

21. Bando H, Zhang C, Takada Y, Yamasaki R, Saito S (1991) Impaired secretion of growth hormone-releasing hormone, growth hormone, and IGF-I in elderly men. Acta Endo Copenh 124:31-36

22. D'Costa A, Lenham JE, Ingram RL, Sonntag WE (1993) Comparison of protein synthesis in brain and peripheral tissue during aging. Relationship to insulin-like growth factor-1 and type 1 IGF receptors. Ann N Y Acad Sci 692:253-255

23. Haselbacher G, Humbel R (1982) Evidence for two species of insulin-like growth factor II (IGF II and big IGF II) in human spinal fluid. Endocrinology 110:1822-1824

24. Barnes CA (1994) Normal aging: regional specific changes in hippocampal synaptic transmission. Trends Neurosci 17:13-18

25. Nitsch R (1993) Transneuronal changes in the lesioned entorhinal-hippocampal system. Hippocampus 3:247-256

26. Lapchak PA, Jenden DJ, Hefti F (1991) Compensatory elevation of acetylcholine synthesis in vivo by cholinergic neurons surviving partial lesions of septohippocampal pathway. J Neurosci 12:4737-4744

27. Stenvers K, Lund PK, Gallagher M (1997) Two deafferenting lesions of the hippocampus produce differential changes in IGF mRNA expression in rats. J Neurosci (submitted)

28. Baxter MG, Bucci DJ, Wiley RG, Gorman LK, Gallagher M (1995) Selective immunotoxic lesions of basal forebrain cholinergic cells: effects on learning and memory in rats. Behav Neurosci 109:714-722

29. Amaral DG, Witter MP (1995) Hippocampal formation. In: Paxinos G (ed) The rat nervous system. Academic Press, New York, pp 443-493

30. Lund PK (1994) Insulin-like growth factors. In: Dockray G, Walsh JH (eds) Gut peptides: Biochemistry and physiology. Raven, New York, pp 587-613

31. Simmons JG, Hoyt EC, Westwick JK, Brenner DA, Pucilowska JB, Lund PK (1995) Insulin-like growth factor-I (IGF-I) and epidermal growth factor (EGF) interact to regulate growth and gene expression in IEC-6 intestinal epithelial cells. Mol Endocrinol 9:1157-1165

32. Merlo GR, Basolo F, Fiore L, Duboc L, Hynes NE (1995) p53-dependent and p53-independent activation of apoptosis in mammary epithelial cells reveal a survival function of EGF and insulin. J Cell Biol 128:1185-1196

33. Lund PK, Zimmerman EM (1996) Insulin-like growth factors and inflammatory disease. In: Goodlaerd R, Wright N (eds) Cytokines and growth factors in gastroenterology. Bailliere's Clin Gastroenterol, vol 10, London, pp 83-96

The Role of IGF-I in Cerebellar Granule Cell Survival and Terminal Differentiation

P. Calissano[1], M. T. Ciotti[1], C. Galli[1], D. Mercanti[1], L. Dus[1], N. Cánu[1], C. Barbato[1], O. V. Vitolo[1], A. Atlante[2], S. Gagliardi[2]

Introduction

Insulin-like growth factor (IGF) I is a pleiotropic agent for the survival and differentiation of different types of nerve cells during development [1]. IGF-I over-expression in transgenic mice induces a marked increase in size and number of neurones in most cerebral areas [2]. The most thorough studies on IGF-I action within the context of brain are those performed in the last decade on cerebellar neuronal populations. In cerebellum, this somatomedin, its receptor and its specific binding proteins are developmentally expressed in such a fashion as to suggest a crucial role in circuit formation [3, 4]. Similar functions have been previously demonstrated or hypothesised for nerve growth factor (NGF) and other growth factors of the neurotrophin family. The action of neuronal growth factors may be exerted either via retrograde transport from target cells to the perikarion of the innervating neuron or, vice versa, via orthograde transport from the innervating neuron to the target cells [5]. The best characterized example of the former case is represented by NGF [6], while IGF-I displays the second type of trophic interaction with target cells [7].

Our research group is engaged in studying the mechanisms through which rat cerebellar granule cells (CGCs) cultured in vitro undergo death via programmed cell death (PCD) or via necrosis according to the treatment to which are they exposed: removal of depolarizing concentrations of KCl generally employed to grow these neurones is accompanied by activation of a cell death program via apoptosis [8, 9]; excessive exposure to the excitatory aminoacid glutamate causes death via necrosis [10]. In both cases the concentration of Ca_i^{2+} plays a crucial role since PCD is initiated [9] by a drop of Ca_i^{2+} while necrosis is due to an excessive influx of this cation via N-methyl-d-aspartate (NMDA) and kainate receptors.

During the course of these studies, we found that IGF-I exerts a dual role on CGCs. On one side it largely prevented apoptosis caused by the KCl shift [8] and, on the other side, it rendered sensitive to the toxic action of glutamate CGCs previously resistant to this excitatory aminoacid [11]. Further studies

[1]Institute of Neurobiology, C.N.R., 00167 Roma, and [2]Centro di Studio dei Mitocondri e Metabolismo Energetico, C.N.R., Bari, Italy

demonstrated that such sensitizing action is due to the increased expression of glutamate receptors and voltage-operated Na^+ channels. This finding led us to hypothesize that IGF-I was endowed with dual actions on CGCs in vitro: a general trophic action which is the consequence of an efficient anti-apoptotic effect, and a more specific up-regulation of glutamate receptors and voltage-operated Na^+ channel subunits [11, 12].

The glutamate-sensitizing activity is not due to a direct effect of IGF-I on the expression of glutamate receptors, but is an indirect consequence of its trophic action that allows the optimum survival of CGCs. The CGCs in turn produce and release in culture a small mol. wt. peptide which appears to be the actual inducer of glutamate receptors and voltage-operated Na^+ channels.

The Anti-Apoptotic Action of IGF-I

CGCs undergo death via apoptosis when deprived of the depolarizing concentrations of KCl (25 mM) usually employed for their survival in culture. In view of the previously documented trophic and glutamate-sensitizing action of IGF-I on these neurones [11], it was hypothesized that this somatomedin exerted its trophic action by antagonizing the apoptotic pathway initiated by KCl removal. IGF-I was the most efficient physiological anti-apoptotic agent acting on CGCs (Fig. 1). During studies aimed at identifying all substances endowed with anti-apoptotic activity, it was found that adenosine is also capable of inhibiting the apoptotic program activated in CGCs by the KCl shift (data not shown). IGF-I and this nucleoside may act in concert or, alternatively, on two distinct neuronal subpopulations of CGCs. It is worth mentioning that, under these conditions, CGCs constitute 95% of the cells present in culture.

The KCl shift from 25 mM to 5 mM triggers apoptosis by selectively closing voltage-operated, L-type Ca^{2+} channels. Several distinct pharmacological experiments demonstrated that the actual triggering of the signal transduction pathway leading to apoptosis was the partial closure of these channels. It was therefore of interest to assess whether the anti-apoptotic action of IGF-I was achieved by counteracting such closure and restoring the normal Ca_i^{2+} concentration. However, IGF-I did not impede the Ca_i^{2+} drop caused by KCl reduction (Fig. 2). Since KCl reduction is the earliest, triggering event of apoptosis, the anti-apoptotic action of IGF-I must be downstream of the Ca_i^{2+} drop and may therefore bypass this event.

How does IGF-I exerts its action? Having established that apoptosis onset requires synthesis of new mRNA and proteins - apparent from the partial inhibition by actinomycin D and cycloheximide, respectively - a series of experiments was carried out to assess the time-course of such syntheses. The rescue time, i.e. the time sufficient to rescue 50% of neurones otherwise doomed to die for a previous exposure to the apoptotic signal, was 6 h if the rescue signal was KCl or IGF-I (Fig. 3). This finding indicates that within 6 h CGCs synthesize killer protein mRNA sufficient to cause death of 50% of the neuronal popula-

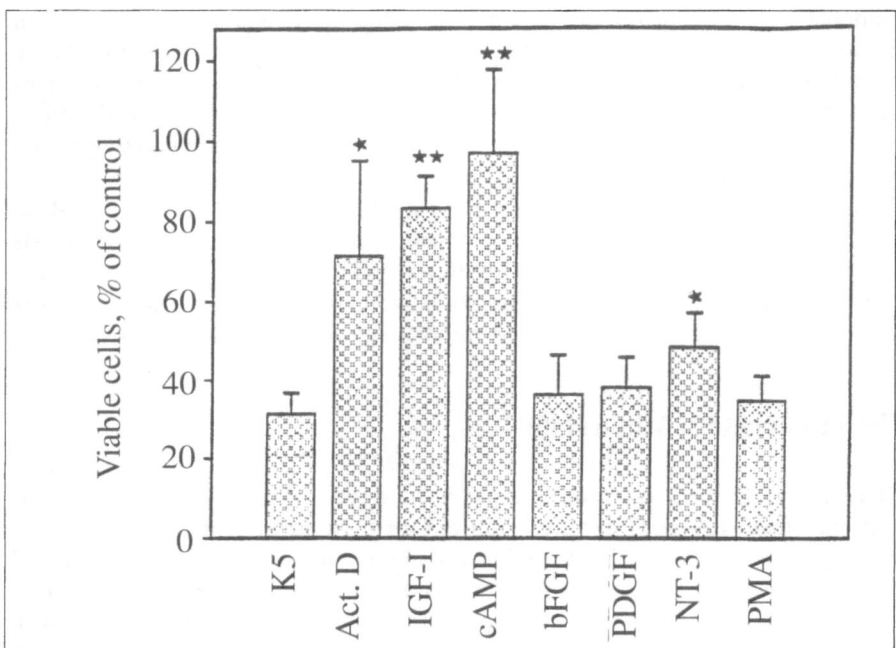

Fig. 1. Survival of neurons after treatment with various agents in low K⁺. Neurons were switched from culture medium containing 10% fetal bovine serum and 25 mM KCl to serum-free medium containing 5 mM K⁺ with no additives (*K5*) or with actinomycin D (*Act. D*, 1 μg/ml), IGF-I (25 ng/ml), forskolin (10 μM; to increase cAMP), bFGF (100 ng/ml), PDGF-A (20 ng/ml), NT-3 (50 ng/ml), or phorbol 12-myristate 13-acetate (*PMA*, 100 nM). Control represents survival in serum-free medium containing 25 mM KCl. Survival was quantified by fluorescein diacetate staining 48 h after treatment. Each bar represents mean ± SD of five randomly chosen microscopic fields taken from three culture dishes. Data are representative of three experiments. Statistically significant differences from K5 were estimated by the Student *t* test: *, *P* < 0.01; **, *P* < 0.001. (From [8])

tion, and that KCl and IGF-I inhibit this process with the same efficacy. As this experimental model provides a large population of CGCs undergoing apoptosis in a relatively marked, synchronous fashion, future studies should allow the identification and cloning of the gene(s) involved in this program of cell death.

   The energetic state of neurones plays an essential role in protecting them from insults of different natures as well from external apoptotic signals. We wished to assess whether the energetic state of CGCs was involved in the early phases of the apoptotic process. Phosphorylative capacity, a significant parameter of energy metabolism, was measured in control neurones and in neurones undergoing apoptosis. The RCR (Respiratory control ratio) value, a measure of the phosphorylative activity of a cell, was reduced 50% within 90-120 min after beginning of apoptosis, indicating that mitochondrial function was rapidly and massively impaired (data not shown). IGF-I, but not IGF-II, was fully effective in preserving the phosphorylative capacity of CGCs even in conditions (5 mM

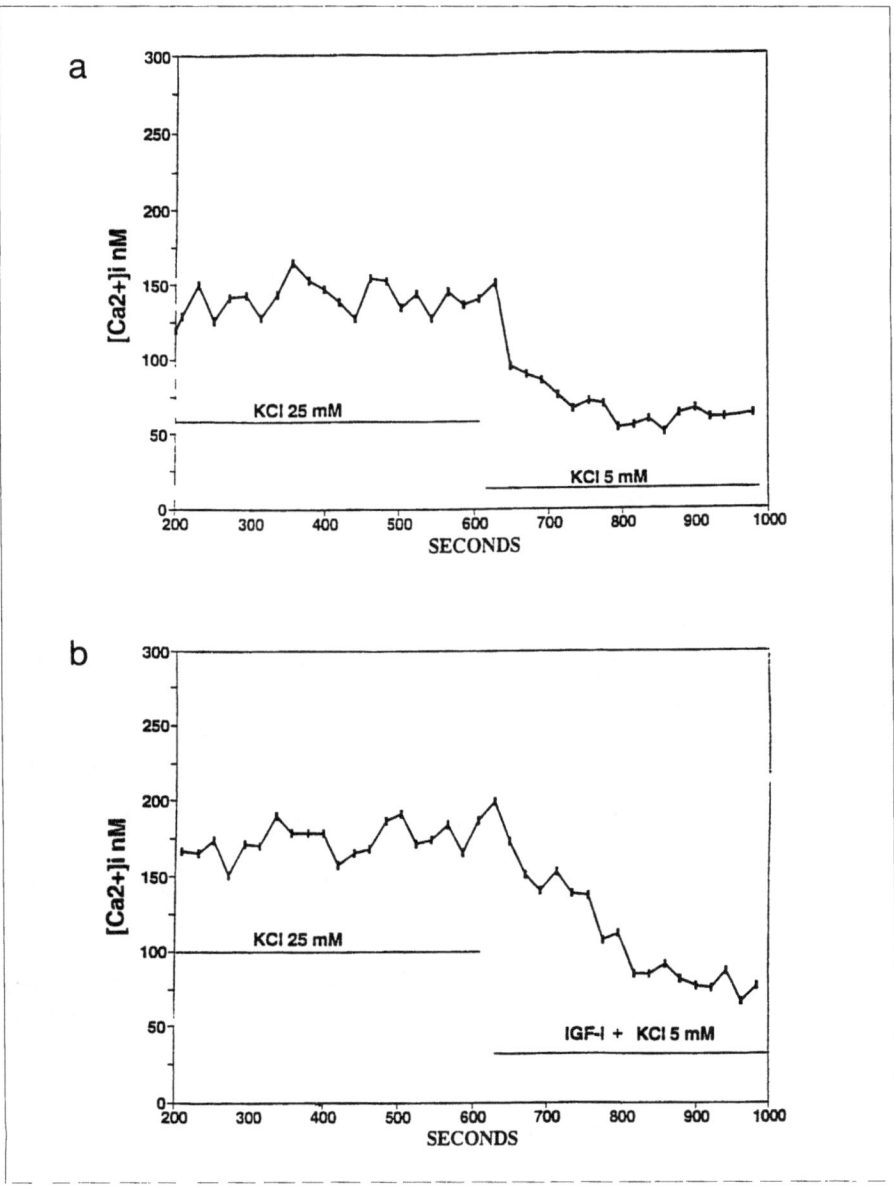

Fig. 2a,b. Rapid change in intracellular $[Ca^{2+}]_i$ induced by lowering extracellular KCl. Neurons grown for 6-7 days in vitro (DIV) in standard culture conditions were kept in 25 mM KCl during the entire procedure of washing, loading with fura-2, and equilibrating. Neurons were shifted to 5 mM KCl with no addition (**a**), or 25 ng/ml IGF-I (**b**). Traces correspond to four samples from different cultures, each representative of 45-60 neurons. (From [9])

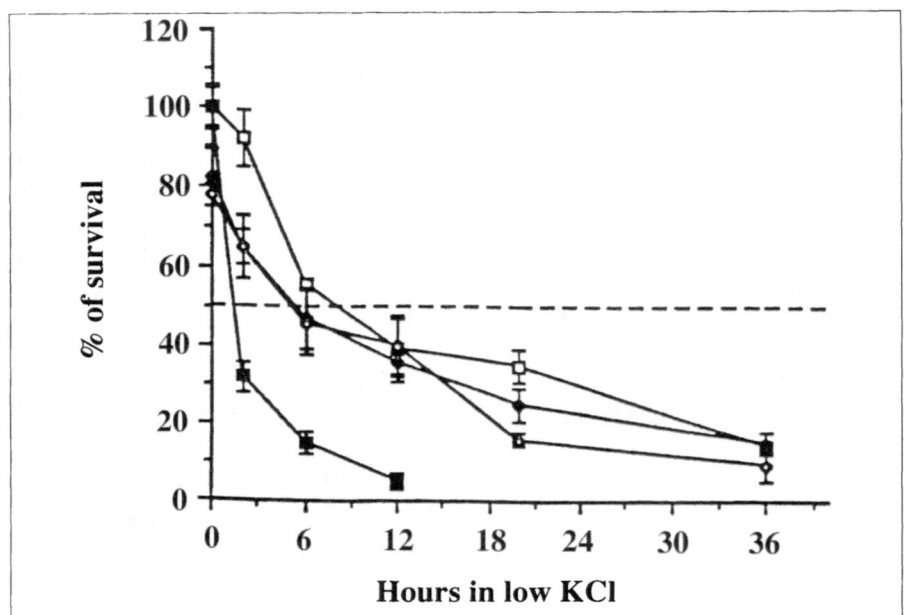

Fig. 3. Commitment point to death of cerebellar granule neurons. Apoptosis was triggered by lowering extracellular KCl from 25 mM to 5 mM. Rescue treatment involved adding high KCl (*open squares*), 10 μM forskolin (*solid diamonds*), 25 ng/ml IGF-I (*open diamonds*), 1 μg/ml actinomycin D (*solid squares*) at the indicated times. Neuronal viability was evaluated by counting intact nuclei 48 h after the initial KCl deprivation. 100% corresponds to the number of neurons susceptible to death after 48 h in 5 mM KCl. Values are expressed as mean ± SD from three separate experiments performed in duplicate. (From [9])

KCl) that caused activation of apoptosis (Fig. 4). This somatomedin was also more efficient than ROS (Reactive Oxygen Species) scavengers such as superoxide dismutase, or antioxidants such as dithiothreitol (DTT), glutathione or vitamin C in counteracting the progressive impairment of mitochondrial function due to onset of programmed cell death (not shown). These findings indicate that IGF-I is the most effective, anti-apoptotic substance tested in CGCs.

IGF-I and Glutamate Sensitivity

Addition of human recombinant IGF-I to cultures of CGCs resistant to glutamate renders these cells sensitive to the toxic action of this excitatory neurotransmitter. This effect is achieved by up-regulation of kainate and NMDA glutamate receptors and by increased expression, or function, of voltage-operated Na^+ channels. This latter effect implies that NMDA toxicity requires the expression of voltage-operated Na^+ channels since their action depends on a concomitant depolarization of the membrane.

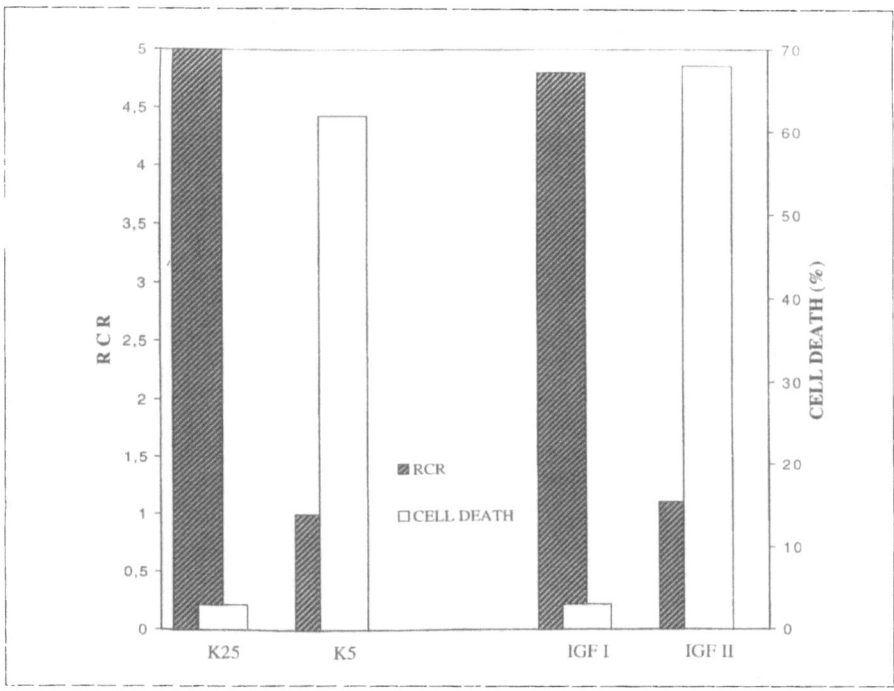

Fig. 4. IGF-I prevents the impairment of cellular respiration. 7 DIV CGCs (15×10^6 per well) in serum-free culture medium were switched from 25 mM KCl (*K25*) to 5 mM KCl (*K5*) in the absence or presence of either IGF-I (25 ng/ml) or IGF-II (25 ng/ml). 8 h later, CGCs were collected, suspended in phosphate-buffered saline, homogenized, and aliquots corresponding to 0.2 mg protein were incubated at 37°C in a water-jacketed glass vessel to monitor polarographically O_2 consumption by succinate either in the absence or presence of ADP. RCR value is reported (*left ordinate*). The extent of cell death determined by counting viable neurons is expressed as the percentage of dead cells versus total viable cells 24 h after switching to low [K^+] (*right ordinate*). The experiment was repeated three times with cell preparations from different groups of animals. Experimental variation was approximately 10%

The action of IGF-I is not achieved "directly" on the synthesis and expression of glutamate receptors but, rather, it is the consequence of a pleiotropic action exerted by IGF-I on CGCs. The sensitivity of these neurones to the toxic action of glutamate is not an invariant property but, on the contrary, varies according to the volume of culture medium in which they are grown [13] (Fig. 5). A 3-fold increase of medium increased the extent of CGCs viable after a 100 μM glutamate pulse from 25% to 80%. When the medium conditioned by CGCs grown in low volume (LV) for 6 days in vitro (DIV) was transferred to sister cultures grown in high volume (HV) the glutamate-dependent cell death after an additional 2 DIV became comparable to that detected in cells grown under LV conditions. Analogous differential sensitivity occurred if, instead of changing volume, the plating cell density was changed (not shown). Therefore, the higher

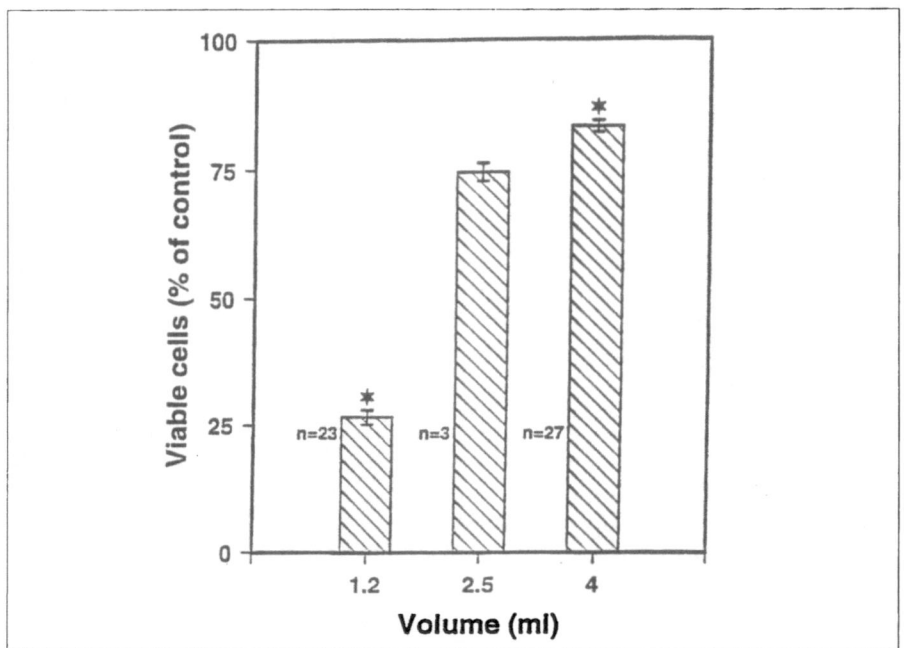

Fig. 5. Effect of different volumes of medium on glutamate sensitivity. Cerebellar granule cells were plated at a density of 2.8×10^5 cells/cm^2 in 12-well clusters (4 cm^2 growth area) and cultured for 8 days in Eagle's basal medium (BME) + 10% fetal bovine serum at the indicated volumes. Values represent mean ± SEM. The number of paired experiments (n) is presented. Student's t test for paired samples indicated a highly significant difference between the data for 1.2 and 4 ml (* $P < 0.0001$). (From [13])

the cell density or the lower the culture medium volume, the greater is the sensitivity to glutamate. If CGCs grown at low density were further incubated with medium conditioned by high density cultures, their glutamate sensitivity was similar to that detectable in neurones plated at high density. These findings led us to hypothesize and demonstrate that cultures of CGCs synthesize and secrete a substance, operationally defined as glutamate-sensitizing activity (GSA), which modulates the functional expression of glutamate receptors. Such sensitizing activity is probably achieved with an autocrine mechanism and is specific for CGCs since medium conditioned by pure glial cells of the same cerebellar source lacked GSA. Moreover, this activity was not effective on GABAergic neurones which represent 2-3% of the cell culture population [13].

We wished to investigate substances which sustained the production of GSA. To this aim, several compounds of different origins were tested. The possibility that such GSA could be attributable to glutamate itself or to some metabolite such as lactate released in culture during the 8 DIV incubation was ruled out with ad hoc experiments [13]. The possibility that NO could be responsible GSA was also ruled out with experiments involving for NO chelators such as haemoglobin or NO producers such as L-nitro-L-arginine methyl ester (NAME). Growth factors such as IGF-I and brain derived neurotrophic factor (BDNF), and hormones such as 3,5,3'-triiodothyronine (T3) were tested in Eagle's basal medium devoid of serum and containing the tested factor. In these experiments, IGF-I was the most effective in sustaining the production and release in culture of GSA [13]. IGF-I supported the production and accumulation of GSA in the culture medium in an amount only slightly lower than that of cells grown in medium containing calf serum. Thus, medium conditioned by CGCs grown with IGF-I markedly increased glutamate sensitivity in a 24 h period of incubation (Fig. 6a). In an analogous experiment performed by adding conditioned medium at 1 DIV and testing the response to glutamate at different periods thereafter, the response of CGCs to glutamate was markedly accelerated (Fig. 6b). Thus, while at 3 and 4 DIV, 70% and 65% of CGCs, respectively, survived the glutamate treatment, only 10-15% of neurones of sister cultures grown in conditioned medium containing serum survived glutamate treatment at 3 and 4 DIV. IGF-I was only partially less effective than fetal bovine serum in sustaining the production of GSA. It is worth considering that serum contains IGF-I and its action in sustaining GSA production could therefore be, at least in part, attributable to this IGF-I pool.

When IGF-I, IGF-II, aFGF, α-TNF or T3 was added to high volume or low density cultures, the glutamate sensitivity after 6 DIV was not substantially different from that of cells grown in serum [13]. This finding indicates that IGF-I and other, less effective trophic substances do not act directly on the cellular production of GSA but, rather, exert a pleiotropic action which is permissive for the production and release in culture of GSA. When the cell mass-to-volume ratio was low, as in low cell density or high volume cultures, neurones survived because of the presence of IGF-I but did not produce enough GSA to induce full glutamate sensitivity. When, on the contrary, IGF-I was added to high cell density or to low volume cultures, its pleiotropic action allowed production of GSA in an amount sufficient to induce the functional expression of glutamate receptors in almost all CGCs. We found that the action of GSA was largely inhibited by actinomycin D (not shown) indicating that it requires transcription [3].

GSA up-regulation of functional expression of glutamate receptors consists, at least in part, in increasing the exposure and probably the synthesis of NMDA receptors. This conclusion is supported by results of MK-801 binding (Fig. 7) to CGCs cultured in conditioned medium containing GSA for different periods, in analogy with the studies of Fig. 6. The binding of this specific NMDA receptor (NMDAR) inhibitor, representing the amount of NMDAR-1 subunit on the surface of CGCs was 150% higher than that of sister cultures grown for 4 DIV in the absence of GSA (Fig. 7a). Only a 60% increase in binding was found if GSA was added at 6 DIV and measured at 8 DIV (Fig. 7b). These findings confirm studies on the glutamate-sensitivity accelerating action of GSA and indicate that this effect is probably due to an increased expression on the cytoplasmic membrane of NMDA receptors and probably of other types of glutamate receptors. This conclusion is supported by experiments measuring NMDA-evoked currents in intact CGCs cultured in the presence or absence of conditioned

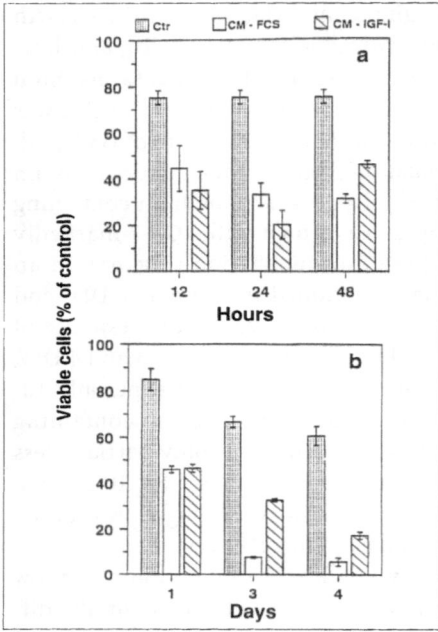

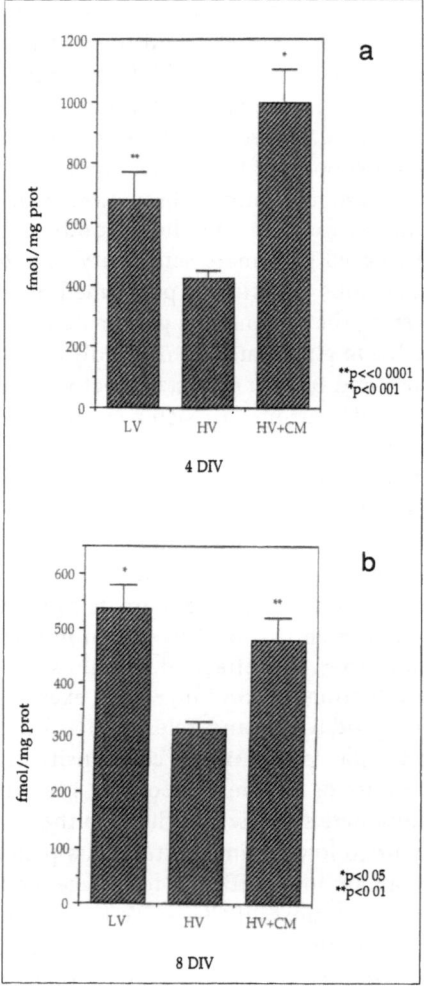

Fig. 6a,b. Time course of the action of conditioned media. **a** Cells were plated in high volume conditions (2.8 x 10^5 cells/cm^2; 4 ml medium in 12-well clusters) and incubated for 6 DIV, after which medium was replaced with conditioned medium derived from low-volume cultures (2.8 x 10^5 cells/cm^2; 2 ml medium in 35 mm dish) grown for 8 days in medium containing fetal bovine serum (*CM-FCS*) or containing human recombinant IGF-I (*CM-IGF-I*). Twelve, 24 and 48 h after the change of medium, cells were tested for glutamate sensitivity. Parallel cultures without a change of medium served as controls (*Ctr*). Values are mean ± SEM of at least three experiments each performed in duplicate (*n* = 7, 7, 21 for the 48 h data). **b** Cells were plated under the high-density condition, and after 1 day of culture the medium was replaced with 8-day conditioned medium (*CM-FCS or CM-IGF-I*). One, 3 and 4 days after the change of medium, cells were tested for glutamate sensitivity (100 μM for 30 min). Sister cultures were grown without any change of medium (control, *Ctr*). Notice the marked accelerating action of conditioned media on the onset of glutamate sensitivity. Values are mean ± SEM of two experiments each performed in duplicate. (From [13])

Fig. 7a,b. MK-801 binding to CGCs cultured in conditioned medium containing GSA. **a** Cells were grown in low volume (*LV*), high volume (*HV*) or high volume, conditioned medium (HV + CM) for 4 DIV. **b** Cells were grown as in **a** but GSA-containing CM was added at 6 DIV and binding was performed at day 8. (From [14])

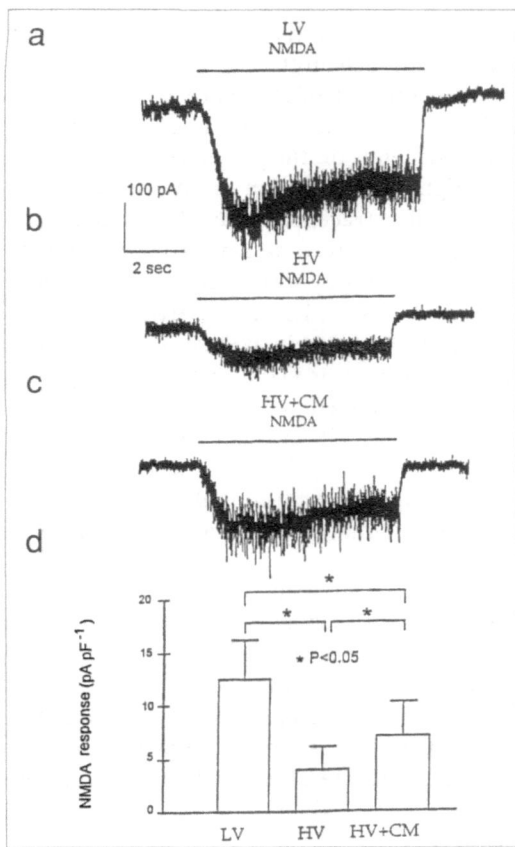

Fig. 8a-d. NMDA-evoked currents in intact CGCs. **a-c** Traces typical of 100 μM NMDA application. **a** Low vol-ume (*LV*) culture conditions. **b** High volume (*HV*). **c** High volume culture conditions for 6 DIV followed by medium replace-ment with GSA-containing condi-tioned medium (*CM*). **d** Average experimental values. (From [14])

medium containing GSA (Fig. 8). GSA added at 6 DIV to cells cultured in high volume conditions increased 30-40% the currents evoked by 100 μM NMDA.

Conclusion

IGF-I is endowed with a general, pleiotropic action on many different types of nerve cells of the central nervous system. This action is well exemplified in cerebellar granule cells cultured in vitro. Removal of depolarizing concentra-tions of KCl immediately unlocked a cell death program which was blocked by addition of IGF-I (or adenosine and its analogues) to cell cultures. In the living animal, neurones require (a) electrical activity assuring sufficient Ca^{2+} entry, or (b) anti-apoptotic action of IGF-I, adenosine or other chemical messengers to prevent PCD activation. The two different stimuli-electrical or chemical-may be alternative or concomitant or may constitute a unique mechanism whereby Ca^{2+} influx triggered by the electrical activity is not devoted to inhibit PCD, but is instrumental to the activation of the exocytotic pathway leading to secretion of IGF-I or adenosine and its analogues. In this case, CGCs would be operating in an autocrine fashion by releasing such an IGF-I pool.

Whatever the source of IGF-I for the control of PCD, it is clear that IGF-I's pleiotropic action is also instrumental for the production and release in culture of GSA. Terminal differentiation of CGCs depends on the presence of depolarizing concentrations of KCl or of IGF-I. High KCl mimics an in vivo situation of electrical activity with consequent influx of extracellular Ca^{2+}. This cation, in turn, either blocks the apoptotic program of these neurones via an as yet unknown pathway, or activates an exocytotic pathway which releases anti-apoptotic substance(s), possibly IGF-I and/or adenosine. IGF-I, in particular, could contribute in a crucial fashion to block PCD. Whether its release is achieved by the Ca^{2+} entry mechanism in an autocrine fashion or via an independent pathway operated by other nerve cells has to be ascertained by in vivo experiments.

The pool of IGF-I released by CGCs, Purkinje cells or other cultured components of the cerebellum allows optimal survival of CGCs which, in turn, synthesize and release in culture a small peptide capable of up-modulating glutamate receptor expression. The acquisition of a glutamatergic phenotype represents the final step of CGC differentiation.

In view of the crucial role played by glutamate receptors, in particular by those of NMDA type, in physiological functions such as learning and memory as well as in pathological conditions associated with reduced oxygen or glucose supply, the identification and characterization of GSA represents an important step for the elucidation of the mechanisms, and possible interventions, modulating the expression of these receptors. IGF-I may support the production of GSA in other cerebral areas and therefore contribute, although indirectly, to the modulation of the glutamatergic system.

Acknowledgements

This work has been carried out under a research contract with NE.FA.C. within the National Research Plan, Neurobiological Systems of the Ministero della Ricerca Scientifica e Tecnologica.

References

1. Hepler JE, Lund PK (1990) Molecular biology of the insulin-like growth factors: relevance to nervous system function. Mol Neurobiol 4:93-127
2. Carson MJ, Beheringer RR, Brinster RL, McMorris FA (1993) Insulin-like growth factor I increases brain growth and central nervous system myelination in transgenic mice. Neuron 10:729-740
3. Zhang W, Lee W-H, Triarhou C (1996) Grafted cerebellar cells in a mouse model of hereditary ataxia express IGF-I system genes and partially restore behavioural function. Nat Med 2:65-71

4. Torres-Aleman I, Pons S, Arevalo MA (1994) The insulin-like growth factor I system in the rat cerebellum; developmental regulation and role in neuronal survival and differentiation. J Neurosci Res 39:117-126
5. Korsching S (1993) The neurotrophic factor concept: a re-examination. J Neurosci 13:2739-2748
6. Levi Montalcini R (1987) The nerve growth factor 37 years later. Science 237:1154-1162
7. Nieto-Bona MP, Garcia-Segura LM, Torres-Aleman I (1993) Orthograde transport of insulin-like growth factor I from the inferior olive to the cerebellum. J Neurosci Res 36:520-527
8. D'Mello SR, Galli C, Ciotti T, Calissano P (1993) Induction of apoptosis in cerebellar granule neurones by low potassium: inhibition of death by insulin-like growth factor 1 and cAMP. Proc Natl Acad Sci USA 90:10989-10993
9. Galli C, Meucci O, Scorziello A, Werge TW, Calissano P, Schettini G (1995) Apoptosis in cerebellar granule cells is blocked by high KCl, forskolin and IGF-1 through distinct mechanisms of action: the involvement of intracellular calcium and RNA synthesis. J Neurosci 15:1172-1179
10. Choi DW (1990) The role of glutamate neurotoxicity in hypoxic-ischemic neuronal death. Annu Rev Neurosci 13:171-182
11. Calissano P, Ciotti MT, Battistini L, Zona C, Angelini A, Merlo D, Mercanti D (1993) Recombinant human insulin-like growth factor I exerts a trophic action and confers glutamate sensitivity on glutamate-resistant cerebellar granule cells. Proc Natl Acad Sci USA 90:8752-8756
12. Zona C, Ciotti MT, Calissano P (1995) Human recombinant IGF-I induces the functional expression of AMPA/kainate receptors in cerebellar granule cells. Neurosci Lett 186:75-78
13. Ciotti MT, Giannetti S, Mercanti D, Calissano P (1996) A glutamate-sensitising activity in conditioned media derived from rat cerebellar granule cells. Eur J Neurosci 8:1591-1600
14. Dus L, Canu N, Zona C, Ciotti MT, Calissano P (1998) NMDA receptor modulation by a conditioned medium derived from rat cerebellar granule cells. Eur J Neurosci (in press)

Regulation of Oligodendrocyte Development and CNS Myelination by IGF-I: Prospects for Disease Therapy

F. A. McMorris, G. S. Vemuri, É. Boyle-Walsh, R. Mewar, M. J. Engleka, G. Lesh

Introduction

Myelin is an innovation that arose relatively recently during evolution, being found only in vertebrates and not in lower taxa. In axons ensheathed by myelin, which forms a series of insulating segments or "internodes" separated by uninsulated nodes of Ranvier, action potentials are conducted in saltatory fashion, jumping from one node of Ranvier to the next without depolarizing the axonal membrane covered by the intervening myelin. As a result, thin myelinated axons can conduct action potentials at the same velocity as much thicker unmyelinated axons, allowing considerable savings in space without sacrificing performance. Moreover, because membrane depolarization and ion flux occur only at the nodes of Ranvier, myelin reduces the energy cost of conduction by a factor of 100 or more. Without the miniaturization and energy efficiency enabled by myelination, the highly complex nervous systems of vertebrates would not be possible. The importance of myelin to neural function is strikingly illustrated by the devastating consequences of demyelination in multiple sclerosis (MS). However, in spite of myelin's fundamental role in nervous system function and its involvement in MS and other human diseases, relatively little is known about the regulation of myelin production by the myelin-forming cells of the central and peripheral nervous systems (CNS and PNS), oligodendrocytes and Schwann cells, respectively. Clarification of these processes would give us a better fundamental understanding of nervous system development and function, and would likely yield information useful in designing therapies to promote remyelination in MS and other myelin diseases.

IGF-I is a Potent Regulator of Oligodendrocyte Development

Using cultures of developing glial cells explanted from neonatal rat cerebrum and maintained in vitro, we found that IGF-I greatly increased the number of oligodendrocytes that developed during a 2-week culture period [1]. As little as 2-5 ng IGF-I/ml doubled the number of oligodendrocytes, and 100 ng IGF-I/ml

The Wistar Institute, Philadelphia, Pennsylvania, USA

increased the number of oligodendrocytes by 6-fold in the presence of 10% serum and by as much as 60-fold in serum-free medium. Type I IGF receptors were detected on oligodendrocytes, identified by the cell surface expression of the myelin-specific lipid galactocerebroside (GC), and on oligodendrocyte precursors, identified by the surface expression of the A2B5 antigen [1]. IGF-II had similar effects on oligodendrocyte development but was 2- to 4-fold less potent, consistent with its lower binding affinity for type I IGF receptors [2, 3]. These results indicated that IGF-I is a potent inducer of oligodendrocyte development, and demonstrated for the first time that IGF-I regulates oligodendrocyte development [1].

We investigated the mechanisms by which IGF-I increases the number of oligodendrocytes that develop in cultures of cells explanted from perinatal rat cerebrum [4]. A2B5-positive oligodendrocyte precursors were purified by fluorescence-activated cell sorting (FACS) and inoculated as single cells into microculture wells. Addition of IGF-I (100 ng/ml) to the culture medium increased the growth rate and the ultimate size of the resulting clones during the 18-day experimental period. Moreover, 75%-80% of the cells in the IGF-I-treated clones differentiated into GC-positive oligodendrocytes, whereas only 25%-30% became oligodendrocytes in the absence of IGF-I. IGF-I did not increase the number of astrocytes, identified by the expression of glial fibrillary acidic protein (GFAP), that developed in the clones. IGF-I appeared to have the greatest effect on growth and differentiation at a stage when the majority of the cells in the clones were at an intermediate stage of development, characterized by the expression of A2B5 and O4 antigens but not GC. Therefore, we tested the effects of IGF-I on O4-positive, GC-negative intermediate precursor cells. IGF-I induced a 2- to 5-fold increase in the number of cells that incorporated ^{3}H-thymidine into their DNA during a 5-hour pulse. Moreover, IGF-I increased the number of FACS-purified O4-positive cells that developed into oligodendrocytes 4-8 days later. Therefore, IGF-I promotes oligodendrocyte development through both the proliferation of oligodendroglial precursor cells and the induction of precursor cells to develop into oligodendrocytes [3-5]. In addition, Barres and her colleagues have shown that IGF-I is a potent survival factor for oligodendrocytes and their precursors [6]. Therefore, IGF-I acts in three different ways to promote the development of oligodendrocytes: as a mitogen, as a differentiation factor, and as a survival factor.

IGF-I Promotes Myelination In Vitro and In Vivo

We investigated whether, in addition to increasing the number of oligodendrocytes, IGF-I induces an increase in the synthesis and accumulation of myelin. We first approached this question in vitro using aggregate cultures, established from 16-day-old fetal rat brains, which contain neurons as well as oligodendrocytes and astrocytes. Cultures treated with IGF-I (100 ng/ml) or high insulin (5000 ng/ml, a concentration at which insulin binds to type I IGF receptors and acts as an IGF analog) contained 35%-80% more oligodendrocytes and 30%-90% more myelin than did controls. These data show that IGF-I regulates myelin synthesis as well as oligodendrocyte development in vitro [7].

We then used a transgenic mouse line that overexpresses IGF-I to investigate whether IGF-I regulates myelination in vivo [8]. By postnatal day 55, when brain growth and myelination are essentially complete in normal mice, the brains of transgenic mice were 55% larger than controls (Fig. 1A). Most or all brain structures appeared to be affected. DNA assays and counting of oligodendrocytes in white and gray matter structures indicated that the number of oligodendrocytes was increased by approximately 25% in the transgenic mouse brains, but the total myelin content was increased by 130% (Fig. 1B). Thus, the increase in myelin content was due primarily to an increase in myelin production per oligodendrocyte [8]. This result is in agreement with our finding, in tissue culture studies, that IGF-I treatment of oligodendrocytes increases the amount of the myelin protein 2',3'-cyclic nucleotide 3'-phosphohydrolase (CNP), and of CNP mRNA, expressed per cell [9]. These findings indicate that IGF-I is a potent inducer of myelination in vivo as well as in vitro [8].

Next, we studied a transgenic mouse line that had greatly reduced circulating and tissue levels of IGF-I due to genetic ablation of growth hormone-producing cells. These mice had smaller brains that contained 50% less myelin than did controls [10]. When we interbred these mice with the IGF-I transgenic mice to restore IGF-I levels to normal, brain weight and brain myelin content were also restored to normal, even in the continued absence of growth hormone (GH) [10]. These findings indicate that IGF-I is required for normal myelination in vivo whereas the role of GH is primarily to maintain adequate IGF-I levels [5, 10].

Thus, in addition to regulating the development of oligodendrocytes by promoting oligodendroglial cell proliferation, differentiation and survival, IGF-I continues to regulate oligodendrocyte function once the cells have developed: it regulates the amount of myelin produced by oligodendrocytes, resulting in overproduction of myelin when IGF-I levels are elevated above normal, and a severe myelin deficit when IGF-I levels are abnormally low [8, 10].

Expression of IGF-I and IGF Binding Proteins by Developing Glial Cells

Although IGF-I and IGF-II and their mRNAs are present in brain both pre- and postnatally, the exact sites of synthesis have not been identified. In situ hybridization readily reveals the expression of IGF-I mRNA in CNS neurons, especially the long-axon projection neurons which are ultimately myelinated by oligodendrocytes [11, 12], and northern blot and nuclease protection assays have shown that IGF-I is also expressed by astrocytes [13, 14]. However, previous studies have failed to detect synthesis of IGFs or IGF mRNAs in oligodendrocytes or their precursors in vivo, perhaps due to limitations in the sensitivity of the methods. Therefore we investigated IGF-I mRNA expression in developing oligodendroglial cells from rat cerebrum using a highly sensitive method, reverse transcriptase-polymerase chain reaction (RT-PCR) [15]. PCR primers were designed to amplify a 296-base sequence of IGF-I mRNA; the amplified sequence spans a 50 kb intron so that any contaminating genomic DNA would not be amplified. PCR-amplified bands were confirmed as IGF-I by molecular weight, hybridization to IGF-I-specific cDNA and antisense oligonucleotide probes, and restriction analysis. At postnatal day 10 (P10), IGF-I mRNA was detected in 0.1 ng total RNA from rat cerebrum, and in RNA samples extracted from as few as 100 cells. Cerebral cells were enzymatically dissociated at P8-P13, and 99%-pure populations of O4-positive or GC-positive cells were isolated by FACS. IGF-I mRNA was detected reproducibly in 100-cell aliquots of O4-positive/GC-negative cells, but was undetectable when the cells became GC-positive oligodendrocytes. Thus, IGFs in the in vivo milieu of developing oligodendroglial cells may be derived from multiple sources: astrocytes and target neurons express IGF-I, choroid plexus and meninges express IGF-II and secrete it into cerebrospinal fluid, and both IGF-I and IGF-II may enter the CNS from the circulation. Additionally, IGF-I is expressed by developing oligodendrocytes themselves, suggesting that oligodendrocyte development is, in part, autoregulated ([15] and references therein).

We also investigated the expression of the six high-affinity IGF binding proteins (IGFBPs) that play an important role in modulating the action of IGF-I and IGF-II. Since IGFBPs have a profound and varied effect on IGF function [16, 17], it is important to establish which IGFBPs are present in oligodendrocytes, oligodendrocyte precursors and surrounding astrocytes. We designed PCR primers and probes specific for each of the six high-affinity IGFBPs to detect their transcripts in cells of the oligodendrocyte lineage [18]. Astrocytes and A2B5-positive/O4-negative, O4-positive/GC-negative, and GC-positive oligodendroglial cells were obtained by immunopanning cultured rat brain cells. RNA from these cells was used for RT-PCR with primers for IGFBPs 1-6. Identity of the PCR bands was confirmed by restriction analysis and hybridization using specific probes. Astrocytes expressed all six IGFBPs. Oligodendrocyte lineage cells expressed IGFBPs 3, 4, 5 and 6 but the pattern of expression changed during development: A2B5-positive precursors expressed IGFBPs 3, 4, 5 and 6, but expression of IGFBP-4 ceased when the cells reached the O4-positive stage. Therefore, intermediate precursors and oligodendrocytes express IGFBPs 3, 5 and 6 but not IGFBP-4 [18]. Although the functional roles of the individual IGFBPs are not fully understood, some differences have been identified. For example, IGFBP-4 is exclusively inhibitory whereas the others can be either stimulatory or inhibitory depending on other factors [16, 17]. IGFBP2, expressed by astrocytes, has been proposed to play a role in oligodendrocyte regeneration by aiding in the presentation of astrocyte-produced IGF-I to receptor-bearing oligodendroglial cells [19]. Expression of IGFBPs by oligodendroglial cells indicates that the cells modulate their own responsiveness to IGF-I. Changes in the pattern of IGFBP expression during development suggests that the nature of this modulation changes qualitatively and quantitatively with development [18].

Prospects for Therapy of Demyelinating Disease with IGF-I

Multiple sclerosis (MS), the most common neurological disorder diagnosed in young adults, is characterized by inflammation and autoimmune demyelination in the CNS [20-24]. Although a small amount of remyelination occurs in MS, most demyelinated axons remain chronically demyelinated [20-30]. Promotion of remyelination is a reasonable strategy for therapy that would be expected to result in significant functional recovery in MS patients, and could potentially be undertaken even without further advances in understanding the etiology or pathogenic mechanisms of the disease [25, 30, 31]. Promotion of remyelination would be expected to be beneficial in other myelin diseases as well. Because of the potent effects of IGF-I in promoting oligodendrocyte development and myelination, it was recognized early on that IGF-I had therapeutic potential for promoting remyelination and clinical improvement in MS and other myelin diseases [1, 31]. More recently, it has been shown that IGF-I promotes remyelination and enhances clinical recovery in rats with experimental autoimmune encephalomyelitis (EAE), an experimental demyelinating disease that resembles MS in many features, as well as in several other experimental demyelinating paradigms [32-35]. Moreover, clinical experience with IGF-I for the treatment of other disorders has demonstrated that IGF-I is well tolerated and safe [36-38]. These considerations suggest that clinical trials with IGF-I for the therapy of MS are justified at this time [31].

Signal Transduction Mechanisms Mediating IGF-I Action in Oligodendrocytes

We have been investigating the signal transduction mechanisms mediating IGF-I action in oligodendrocytes to understand the regulatory pathways leading to the different IGF-I responses in oligodendroglial cells (proliferation, differentiation, survival, and myelin synthesis) and to understand how IGF-I activates these pathways at different times during oligodendrocyte development. Such information will prove useful in understanding how oligodendrocyte development is regulated, and may be valuable in developing therapies to target specific cellular responses while avoiding unwanted side-effects.

Studies with the IGF-I receptor and the homologous insulin receptor have shown that upon activation these receptors tyrosine-phosphorylate the intracellular docking proteins IRS-1 (insulin receptor substrate-1), IRS-2, Gab1 (Grb2 binder-1), Shc, and possibly the recently-described IRS-3 [39-43]. Phospho-rylated Shc binds and activates the adapter molecule Grb2, which then activates the Ras-Raf-MAP kinase pathway leading ultimately to cell proliferation and changes in gene activity. The IRS proteins and Gab1 have multiple tyrosines which, when phosphorylated, serve as sites for binding and activating numerous downstream signaling partners, including Grb2, phosphatidylinositol

3-kinase (PI3-K), SHP-2 [37, 38, 42], phospholipase-Cγ (PLCγ) [38, 40], Nck, Fyn [39, 45], and probably other, as yet unidentified, signaling partners. Each of these molecules activates additional downstream signal transduction molecules leading ultimately to biological responses including DNA synthesis, cell proliferation, changes in gene activity, differentiation, survival, glucose transport, vesicle trafficking, secretion, cytoskeletal changes and motility [39].

We investigated the role of PI3-K in the various responses of oligodendrocytes to IGF-I. Wortmannin and LY294002, two specific and potent inhibitors of PI3-K, caused 60%-70% of cells to initiate cell death processes within 24 h, as quantitated by an MTT tetrazolium assay for surviving cells and by measurement of DNA content [44]. Similar results were observed with oligodendrocyte precursor cells and with mature oligodendrocytes. To determine whether DNA in the dying cells was undergoing fragmentation, a characteristic of apoptotic death, we performed terminal deoxynucleotide transferase (TdT)-mediated dUTP-biotin nick end-labeling (TUNEL) assays. In the presence of wortmannin, 20% of the cells became TUNEL-positive within 4 h (as compared to 3% of control cells), before any significant differences could be detected in glucose transport or in cell viability as measured by the MTT tetrazolic assay. By 24 h, 60%-65% of the cells were TUNEL-positive. Cell death due to wortmannin (Fig. 2) or LY294002 (data not shown) could not be prevented by addition of the oligodendrocyte survival factors IGF-I, neurotrophin-3 (NT-3), platelet-derived growth factor (PDGF), basic fibroblast growth factor (bFGF), ciliary neurotrophic factor (CNTF), N-acetyl cysteine, vitamin C, vitamin E, progesterone or serum, singly or in various combinations. We concluded that oligodendrocyte survival, in the absence or presence of exogenous oligodendroglial cell survival factors or serum, depends on a PI3-K-dependent signaling pathway. Inhibition of this critical enzyme activity induces apoptosis, resulting in cell death [46].

Although four (or possibly five [43]) docking proteins are known to mediate signals from the IGF-I and insulin receptors, nothing is known about which proteins perform these functions in oligodendrocytes. Therefore we investigated the expression of docking proteins in developing oligodendrocytes. By RT-PCR analysis of cell populations highly purified by immunopanning, we found that IRS-1 is expressed in oligodendroglial cells in all developmental stages examined: in A2B5-positive oligodendrocyte precursors, in O4-positive/GC-negative intermediate precursors and in GC-positive oligodendrocytes. In western blotting experiments conducted in collaboration with Drs. Albert Wong and Marina Holgado-Madruga, we found that both precursors and GC-positive oligodendrocytes also express Gab1 [47, 48]. Next, we used immunofluorescence staining and confocal microscopy to examine the expression of IRS-1, IRS-2, Gab1 and Shc, and found that all four are expressed in oligodendroglial cells in each of the developmental stages examined [47, 48]. All four docking proteins are expressed in perinuclear cytoplasm and in the cytoplasmic processes of the cells [47, 48].

We then examined whether IGF-I signals to PI3-K in oligodendroglia via

IRS-1, IRS-2 and/or Gab1, all of which contain consensus docking sites for the p85 regulatory subunit of PI3-K. When oligodendroglial cells were homogenized and cell extracts were immunoprecipitated with antibodies specific to IRS-1, IRS-2 or Gab1, we detected PI3-K activity in all immunoprecipitates, indicating that PI3-K associates with each of the docking proteins in oligodendroglial cells [48, 49]. Similar results were observed with mature (GC-positive) oligodendrocytes and with immature (A2B5-positive, O4-negative) oligodendrocyte precursors. Incubation of oligodendrocyte precursors with IGF-I for 10 min prior to lysis resulted in a 3- to 4-fold increase in PI3-K activity associated with all three docking proteins. In contrast, when oligodendrocytes were tested, IGF-I caused a 3- to 4-fold increase in the amount of PI3-K activity associated with IRS-1 and Gab1, but no change in PI3-K activity associated with IRS-2. Thus, IGF-I activates PI3-K signaling via three different routes in oligodendrocyte precursors, but only two of these three routes are activated by IGF-I in oligodendrocytes [46, 47]. Further information on the IGF-I signaling pathways in developing oligodendrocytes may help explain why IGF-I elicits different responses at different stages of development.

There is extensive overlap in the signaling partners activated by IRS-1, IRS-2 and Gab1: experiments in other systems have shown that all three bind and activate Grb2, PI3-K, SHP-2 and PLCγ, and possibly other signaling intermediates [39-42]. To examine the role of IRS-1, we studied myelination in "knockout" mice in which the irs-1 gene had been inactivated by gene targeting [50], in collaboration with Dr. Ronald Kahn and colleagues at Harvard University [51, 52]. Analyses at ages 14-55 days revealed a deficit of approximately 25%-30% in myelin content in mutant mouse brains (Table 1) [51, 52]. Therefore, in spite of the considerable functional overlap between IRS-1, IRS-2 and Gab1, IRS-1 plays an essential role in normal myelination; the other docking proteins cannot fully compensate for the absence of IRS-1. On the other hand, partial compensation does occur, as evidenced by the presence of a partial complement of myelin in the irs-1 knockout mice [51, 52].

Fyn, a non-receptor protein tyrosine kinase of the Src family, may play a role in myelination by transducing signals from myelin-associated glycoprotein (MAG) [53]. This observation implies that MAG may have a previously unrecog-

Table 1. Myelin content in brains of IRS-1 (-/-) and control mice (from [49, 50])

Age (days)	Mean myelin content ± SEM (mg/g)[a]		IRS-1 (-/-), % of control
	IRS-1 (+/+)	IRS-1 (-/-)	
14	8.5 ± 0.6	5.8 ± 0.7	68.1 ± 9.0
43	23.7 ± 1.1	17.8 ± 0.7	75.3 ± 4.6
55	20.6 ± 1.7	15.3 ± 2.1	74.2 ± 11.7

At the indicated ages, brains were removed and weighed; myelin was purified, lyophilized and weighed. For each time point, 3-6 control and 3-5 knockout mouse brains were analyzed.
[a] Data are expressed in milligrams myelin (dry weight) per gram brain (wet weight)

nized receptor function. Fyn may also be involved in other signaling networks of relevance to oligodendrocyte development and function [54, 55]. A recent report that Fyn can dock directly on IRS-1 [45] suggests a role for Fyn in IGF-I signaling as well.

We used immunofluorescence staining and confocal microscopy to investigate Fyn expression, and found that Fyn is highly expressed in oligodendroglial cells at the early precursor, intermediate precursor and mature stages [47, 56, 57]. Fyn appears to be expressed at similar levels at all three developmental stages, suggesting that it is equally important throughout this period. Expression of Fyn is restricted primarily to the cell soma [47, 57]. We also studied the two closely-related kinases Src and Yes and found similar patterns of expression: all three kinases are expressed in oligodendrocytes at the same developmental stages and in approximately the same subcellular locations [47, 57].

To investigate the role of Fyn in the myelination process in vivo, we measured the myelin content of *fyn⁻* knockout mouse brains. Myelin was isolated, lyophilized, and weighed from whole brain of homozygous *fyn⁻* mutants and controls. Average total brain myelin content of the *fyn⁻* mutants was only 34%-57% of control values at postnatal days 15-95, whereas average total brain weight was 67%-74% of controls [47, 56, 57]. Normalized for brain weight, the myelin content of the knockout brains was 47%-77% of controls (Table 2), indicating an essential role for Fyn in myelination [47, 56, 57]. Thus, similar to our experiments with the IRS-1 knockouts, the experiments with Fyn knockout mice show that Fyn plays an essential role in normal CNS myelination and that

Table 2. Myelin content of brains of Fyn (-/-) and control mice (from [47, 56, 57])

Age (days)	Mean myelin content ± SEM (mg/g)[a]		Fyn (-/-), % of control
	Fyn (+/+)	Fyn (-/-)	
15	4.1 ± 0.4	3.1 ± 0.4	76.8 ± 12.5
26	11.8 ± 0.9	5.6 ± 1.0	47.3 ± 8.9
55	26.3 ± 0.9	17.3 ± 0.7	65.8 ± 3.3
95	25.1 ± 1.5	16.3 ± 0.6	65.2 ± 4.7

Animals were killed at the ages indicated, brains were weighed, and myelin was purified, lyophilized and weighed. For each time point, 6-9 control and 6-10 knockout mouse brains were analyzed
[a]Data are expressed in milligrams myelin (dry weight) per gram brain (wet weight)

the closely-related kinases Src and Yes are not able to fully compensate for the absence of Fyn. However, partial compensation does occur, perhaps by Src, Yes or some other, as yet undetermined, process.

Conclusions

IGF-I is a potent regulator of oligodendrocyte development and myelination in the CNS. IGF-I promotes oligodendrocyte development by acting as a mitogen, a differentiation factor and a survival factor. Further, once oligodendrocytes have developed and reached their target axons, IGF-I regulates the amount of myelin they produce. IGF-I deficiency in vivo results in hypomyelination, while IGF-I excess leads to substantial overproduction of myelin. These observations suggest that IGF-I is a good candidate as a therapeutic agent to promote remyelination in MS and other diseases of myelin. IGF-I-induced remyelination may produce significant clinical benefits to patients. Studies on signal transduction mechanisms reveal that IGF-I signaling in oligodendrocytes involves a complex array of signaling molecules with overlapping but non-redundant activities. Further elucidation of these mechanisms and pathways will clarify how IGF-I action and oligodendrocyte development and function are controlled, and may make it possible to refine therapies based on IGF-I so as to target desired biological responses and leave others unaffected.

Acknowledgements

This work was supported by grants 32394 and 32122 from the National Institutes of Health, grants from the National Multiple Sclerosis Society, and a grant from the H.H. Smith Foundation.

References

1. McMorris FA, Smith TM, DeSalvo S, Furlanetto RW (1986) Insulin-like growth factor I/somatomedin C: A potent inducer of oligodendrocyte development. Proc Natl Acad Sci USA 83:822-826
2. McMorris FA, Furlanetto RW (1989) Insulin-like growth factor II induces development of oligodendrocytes from rat brain. The Endocrine Society, 71st Annual Meeting, A603
3. McMorris FA, Furlanetto RW, Mozell RL, Carson MJ, Raible DW (1990) Regulation of oligodendrocyte development by insulin-like growth factors and cyclic nucleotides. Ann N Y Acad Sci 605:101-109
4. McMorris FA, Dubois-Dalcq M (1988) Insulin-like growth factor I promotes cell proliferation and oligodendroglial commitment in rat glial progenitor cells developing in vitro. J Neurosci Res 21:199-209
5. McMorris FA, Mozell RL, Carson MJ, Shinar Y, Meyer RD, Marchetti N (1993) Regulation of oligodendrocyte development and central nervous system myelination by insulin-like growth factors. Ann N Y Acad Sci 692:321-334
6. Barres BA, Hart IK, Coles HSR, Burne JF, Voyvodic JT, Richardson WD, Raff MC (1992) Cell death and control of cell survival in the oligodendrocyte lineage. Cell 70:31-46
7. Mozell RL, McMorris FA (1991) Insulin-like growth factor I stimulates oligodendrocyte

development and myelination in rat brain aggregate cultures. J Neurosci Res 30:382-390

8. Carson MJ, Behringer RR, Brinster RL, McMorris FA (1993) Insulin-like growth factor I increases brain growth and central nervous system myelination in transgenic mice. Neuron 10:729-740

9. Meyer RD, Marchetti N, McMorris FA (1993) IGF-I increases CNP activity and mRNA per oligodendrocyte. Trans Am Soc Neurochem 24:261

10. Carson M, Behringer RR, Mathews LS, Palmiter RD, Brinster RL, McMorris FA (1989) Hypomyelination caused by growth hormone deficiency is reversed by insulin-like growth factor I in transgenic mice. Trans Am Soc Neurochem 20:286

11. Bartlett WP, Li XS, Williams M, Benkovic S (1991) Localization of insulin-like growth factor-1 mRNA in murine central nervous system during postnatal development. Dev Biol 147:239-250

12. Bondy CA (1991) Transient IGF-I gene expression during the maturation of functionally related central projection neurons. J Neurosci 11:3442-3455

13. Ballotti R, Nielsen FC, Pringle N, Kowalski A, Richardson WD, Van Obberghen E, Gammeltoft S (1987) Insulin-like growth factor I in cultured rat astrocytes: expression of the gene, and receptor tyrosine kinase. EMBO J 6:3633-3639

14. Rotwein P, Burgess SK, Milbrandt JD, Krause JE (1988) Differential expression of insulin-like growth factor genes in rat central nervous system. Proc Natl Acad Sci USA 85:265-269

15. Shinar Y, McMorris FA (1995) Developing oligodendroglia express mRNA for insulin-like growth factor I, a regulator of oligodendrocyte development. J Neurosci Res 42:516-527

16. Kelley KM, Oh Y, Gargosky SE, Gucev Z, Matsumoto T, Hwa V, Ng L, Simpson DM, Rosenfeld RG (1996) Insulin-like growth factor-binding proteins (IGFBPs) and their regulatory dynamics. Int J Biochem Cell Biol 28:619-637

17. LeRoith D (1996) Insulin-like growth factor receptors and binding proteins. Baillieres Clin Endocrinol Metab 10:49-73

18. Mewar R, McMorris FA (1997) Expression of insulin-like growth factor binding protein messenger RNAs in developing rat oligodendrocytes and astrocytes. J Neurosci Res (in press)

19. Liu X, Yao DL, Bondy CA, Brenner M, Hudson LD, Zhou J, Webster HD (1994) Astrocytes express insulin-like growth factor-I (IGF-I) and its binding protein, IGFBP-2, during demyelination induced by experimental autoimmune encephalomyelitis. Mol Cell Neurosci 5:418-430

20. McFarlin DE, McFarland HF (1982) Multiple sclerosis (first of two parts). N Engl J Med 307:1183-1188

21. McFarlin DE, McFarland HF (1982) Multiple sclerosis (second of two parts). N Engl J Med 307:1246-1251

22. McKhann GM (1982) Multiple sclerosis. Annu Rev Neurosci 5:219-239

23. Raine CS (1990) Multiple sclerosis: immunopathologic mechanisms in the progression and resolution of inflammatory demyelination. Res Publ Assoc Res Nerv Ment Dis 68:37-54

24. Waksman BH (1989) Multiple sclerosis. Curr Opin Immunol 1:733-739

25. Prineas JW, Connell F (1979) Remyelination in multiple sclerosis. Ann Neurol 5:22-31

26. Prineas JW, Kwon EE, Goldenberg PZ, Ilyas AA, Quarles RH, Benjamins JA, Sprinkle TJ (1989) Multiple sclerosis. Oligodendrocyte proliferation and differentiation in fresh lesions. Lab Invest 61:489-503

27. Prineas JW, Kwon EE, Goldenberg PZ, Cho ES, Sharer LR (1990) Interaction of

astrocytes and newly formed oligodendrocytes in resolving multiple sclerosis lesions. Lab Invest 63:624-636

28. Ludwin SK (1980) Chronic demyelination inhibits remyelination in the central nervous system. An analysis of contributing factors. Lab Invest 43:382-387

29. Raine CS, Scheinberg LC (1988) On the immunopathology of plaque development and repair in multiple sclerosis. J Neuroimmunol 20:189-201

30. Raine CS, Moore GR, Hintzen R, Traugott U (1988) Induction of oligodendrocyte proliferation and remyelination after chronic demyelination. Relevance to multiple sclerosis. Lab Invest 59:467-476

31. McMorris FA, McKinnon RD (1996) Regulation of oligodendrocyte development and CNS myelination by growth factors: prospects for therapy of demyelinating disease. Brain Pathol 6:313-329

32. Yao DL, Liu X, Hudson LD, Webster HD (1995) Insulin-like growth factor I treatment reduces demyelination and up-regulates gene expression of myelin-related proteins in experimental autoimmune encephalomyelitis. Proc Natl Acad Sci USA 92:6190-6194

33. Liu X, Yao DL, Webster HD (1995) Insulin-like growth factor I treatment reduces clinical deficits and lesion severity in acute demyelinating experimental autoimmune encephalomyelitis. Mult Scler 1:2-9

34. Yao DL, West NR, Bondy CA, Brenner M, Hudson LD, Zhou J, Collins GH, Webster HD (1995) Cryogenic spinal cord injury induces astrocytic gene expression of insulin-like growth factor I and insulin-like growth factor binding protein 2 during myelin regeneration. J Neurosci Res 40:647-659

35. Yao DL, Liu X, Hudson LD, Webster HD (1996) Insulin-like growth factor-I given subcutaneously reduces clinical deficits, decreases lesion severity and upregulates synthesis of myelin proteins in experimental autoimmune encephalomyelitis. Life Sci 58:1301-1306

36. Bondy CA, Underwood LE, Clemmons DR, Guler HP, Bach MA, Skarulis M (1994) Clinical uses of insulin-like growth factor I. Ann Intern Med 120:593-601

37. Vaught JL, Contreras PC, Miller M, Neff N (1998) Neurobiology of rhIGF-I: rationale for use in motor neuron disease. In: Müller EE (ed) IGFs in the Neurons System. Springer-Verlag, Berlin Heidelberg New York, pp 105-114

38. Silani V, Brioschi A, Sampietro A, Ciammola A, Pizzuti A, Scarlato G (1998) rhIGF-I for the treatment of neuromuscular disorders. In: Müller EE (ed) IGFs in the Neurons System. Springer-Verlag, Berlin Heidelberg New York, pp 115-126

39. White MF, Kahn CR (1994) The insulin signaling system. J Biol Chem 269:1-4

40. Holgado-Madruga M, Emlet DR, Moscatello DK, Godwin AK, Wong AJ (1996) A Grb2-associated docking protein in EGF- and insulin-receptor signalling. Nature 379:560-564

41. Sun XJ, Wang LM, Zhang Y, Yenush L, Myers MG Jr, Glasheen E, Lane WS, Pierce JH, White MF (1995) Role of IRS-2 in insulin and cytokine signalling. Nature 377:173-177

42. Sun XJ, Pons S, Wang LM, Zhang Y, Yenush L, Burks D, Myers MG Jr, Glasheen E, Copeland NG, Jenkins NA, Pierce JH, White MF (1997) The IRS-2 gene on murine chromosome 8 encodes a unique signaling adapter for insulin and cytokine action. Mol Endocrinol 11:251-262

43. Lavan BE, Lane WS, Lienhard GE (1997) The 60-kDa phosphotyrosine protein in insulin-treated adipocytes is a new member of the insulin receptor substrate family. J Biol Chem 272:11439-11443

44. Waters SB, Pessin JE (1996) Insulin receptor substrate 1 and 2 (IRS1 and IRS2): what a tangled web we weave. Trends Cell Biol 6:1-3

45. Sun XJ, Pons S, Asano T, Myers MG Jr, Glasheen E, White MF (1996) The Fyn tyrosine kinase binds IRS-1 and forms a distinct signaling complex during insulin action. J Biol Chem 271:10583-10587

46. Vemuri GS, McMorris FA (1996) Oligodendrocytes and their precursors require phosphatidylinositol 3-kinase signaling for survival. Development 122:2529-2537

47. Boyle-Walsh É, Vemuri GS, Holgado-Madruga M, Wong AJ, McMorris FA (1997) Expression of IGF-I signalling molecules in developing rat oligodendrocytes. J Neurochem 69:S9A

48. Vemuri GS, Boyle-Walsh É, Holgado-Madruga M, Engleka MJ, Wong AJ, McMorris FA (1997) Insulin-like growth factor I signals to phosphatidylinositol 3-kinase through the receptor docking proteins IRS-1, IRS-2 and Gab1 in developing oligodendroglial cells. (Manuscript in preparation)

49. Vemuri GS, Boyle-Walsh É, Holgado-Madruga M, Engleka MJ, Wong AJ, McMorris FA (1997) Association of phosphatidylinositol 3-kinase with insulin-like growth factor receptor docking proteins in oligodendroglial cells. J Neurochem 69:S9B

50. Araki E, Lipes MA, Patti ME, Bruning JC, Haag B, Johnson RS, Kahn CR (1994) Alternative pathway of insulin signalling in mice with targeted disruption of the IRS-1 gene. Nature 372:186-190

51. Engleka M, Folli F, Winnay J, Kahn CR, McMorris FA (1996) Insulin-receptor substrate-1 is required for normal myelination. J Neurochem 66:S20A

52. Boyle-Walsh É, Engleka M, Vemuri GS, Holgado-Madruga M, Wiemelt AP, Folli F, Winnay J, Kahn CR, Wong AJ, McMorris FA (1997) Expression of IGF-I signalling molecules in developing rat oligodendrocytes. (Manuscript in preparation)

53. Umemori H, Sato S, Yagi T, Aizawa S, Yamamoto T (1994) Initial events of myelination involve Fyn tyrosine kinase signalling. Nature 367:572-576

54. Maness PF (1992) Nonreceptor protein tyrosine kinases associated with neuronal development. Dev Neurosci 14:257-270

55. Kypta RM, Goldberg Y, Ulug ET, Courtneidge SA (1990) Association between the PDGF receptor and members of the src family of tyrosine kinases. Cell 62:481-492

56. Boyle-Walsh E, Engleka M, Mewar R, Chen J, Stein P, McMorris FA (1996) Detection and cloning of proteins in developing brain that interact with Fyn tyrosine kinase. J Neurochem 66:S87D

57. Boyle-Walsh É, Engleka M, Lesh G, Stein P, McMorris FA (1997) Role of the Src-family protein tyrosine kinases Fyn, Src and Yes in oligodendrocyte development and myelination in vitro and in vivo (in preparation)

IGF-I and Glycosaminoglycans Improve Peripheral Nerve Regeneration and Motor Neuron Survival in Models of Motor Neuron Disease

A. Gorio, L. Vergani, M. Losa, G. Pezzoni, L. Calvano, C. Finco, A. M. Di Giulio, A. Torsello, E. E. Müller

Introduction

The discovery of agents capable of modulating neuronal survival and regeneration has been of interest to scientists since the early days of neuroscience. Recently, research into such agents has greatly increased due to their potential therapeutic use in neurodegenerative disorders [1]. Research related to nervous system regeneration following injury was strongly influenced by studies of Ramon Y Cajal [2] and Tello [3], and by the consolidation of the neuron theory. Tello wrote that lesioned nerves regenerate by forming sprouts which elongate, crossing the site of injury and regrowing into the distal stump up to the denervated muscle. He suggested that the processes of nerve regrowth and muscle reinnervation were promoted by some unknown substance liberated by the distal stump and/or by the denervated muscle. A tremendous advancement in this field came with the work of Levi Montalcini, Hamburgher and Cohen. Their contribution was dual: the description of neuronal death during embryonic development and the discovery of nerve growth factor [4-6]. It is now well known that at least for certain neuronal populations the process of cell death is regulated by the availability of a target-derived trophic factor. Nerve growth factor was the first of such trophic agents characterized [6]. Later it was found that the mammalian salivary gland, which corresponds to the snake venom gland, contained large amounts of nerve growth factor, and it became the most important source of the trophic factor [7]. With sufficient quantities of purified factor available, this field of research increased greatly. Several other neuronal trophic factors were discovered later; their availability was markedly augmented by recombinant DNA technology which supplied enough active substance to allow clinical studies in humans. The concept that particular proteins control neuronal development and function and, thus, have potential therapeutic use was acknowledged by the 1986 Nobel prize for medicine to Levi Montalcini and Cohen for their discovery and investigations of NGF.

Among the factors having trophic effects on the nervous system is insulin-

Laboratories for Research on Pharmacology of Neurodegenerative Disorders and Neuroendocrinology, Department of Medical Pharmacology, University of Milan, Via Vanvitelli 32, 20129 Milan, Italy

like growth factor (IGF) I, though its appreciation as a neurotrophic factor is recent since early work was focused on its metabolic and growth-promoting activities. IGFs were discovered when non-suppressible insulin-like activity was still present in serum after exposure to anti-insulin antibodies. Various semi-purified preparations having both insulin-like effects and growth-promoting activity were named somatomedins [8]. The aminoacid sequence revealed that somatomedins were members of the insulin gene family; thereby they were renamed insulin-like growth factors. Both IGFs and their type I and type II receptors were found in brain and spinal cord [9-11], suggesting a role for IGFs in the nervous system. In vitro studies showed that supplementation of IGFs to culture medium promoted neurite formation and increased survival of sympathetic and sensory peripheral neurons and central neurons [12-14]. The beneficial effects of IGF-I were also observed after in vivo administration in which IGF-I was supplied locally to the muscle or lesion site of the sciatic nerve. Such treatment stimulated intramuscular motor nerve sprouting or sciatic nerve regeneration, respectively [15, 16]. Administration of IGF-I at 1 mg/kg via subcutaneous route reduced forelimb muscle atrophy and loss of strength in *wobbler* mouse motor neuron disease [17].

In our study, in addition to the effects induced by IGF-I, we have also evaluated those of glycosaminoglycans (GAGs) since recent reports have suggested that these agents are active on axonal growth and nerve regeneration [18-20], and that they may regulate the interaction between IGF-I and the insulin-like growth factor binding proteins (IGFBPs) [21, 22].

Animal Models and Experimental Methods

A potentially useful drug for motoneuron disease should have at least four features: 1) enhancement of motoneuron survival; 2) enhancement of motor neuron sprouting and regeneration; 3) prevention of muscle atrophy; and 4) systemic bioavailability. We used three experimental models to assess the therapeutic potential of IGF-I and GAGs in motoneuron disease: the *wobbler* mouse, the *Mnd* mouse, and the neonatal rat subjected to axotomy-induced retrograde degeneration of motor neurons.

The *wobbler* mouse displays forelimb muscle weakness by the age of 3 weeks, accompanied by progressive loss of strength, altered paw positioning and reduced running speed. The forelimb biceps brachii undergo progressive denervation atrophy with motoneuron death and atrophy of musculocutaneous nerve fibers [23]. Upon diagnosis (3 weeks of age) *wobbler* mice were treated for 3 weeks with daily subcutaneous injections of IGF-I or GAGs at the dose of 0.02 mg/kg or 1 mg/kg body weight, respectively. During treatment, animals were weekly subjected to behavioral trials for evaluating forelimb muscle function. The tests consisted in forelimb grip strength and holding time, and running time assessed according to Mitsumoto et al. [24] and Vergani et al. [25]. Holding time measures the time that a mouse can hold onto the edge of a 45°

inclined platform. Running time is that taken to run a distance of 10 cm. At the end of treatment, biceps muscle fiber size, distribution and innervation were measured by classical histology and combined acetylcholinesterase (AChE)-silver staining techniques, respectively, as previously described [26, 27]. Motor neuron survival was evaluated in the biceps brachii by retrograde labeling after injection of horseradish peroxidase coupled to β-cholera toxin (βCht-HRP).

The *Mnd* mouse develops late-onset motoneuron degeneration that is fatal at 10-12 months of age. There is progressive paralysis and loss of strength in the hind limbs associated with changes in neurofilament distribution and accumulation of ubiquitin in the cell bodies [23, 28]. *Mnd* mice were treated daily with 0.02 mg IGF-I or with 1 mg GAGs per kilogram body weight starting at the 150th day of life. Drug treatment ended at postnatal day 300 when the extensor digitorum longus (EDL) muscle and relative nerve were dissected to assess indirect isometric tension of the muscle as previously described [20].

Retrograde degeneration was induced by axotomy in 3-day-old rats by sciatic nerve crush. This lesion causes progressive atrophy of fast muscles, such as the EDL, with poor muscle reinnervation and severe loss of axotomized motor neurons [29]. EDL muscle reinnervation was evaluated by measuring isometric tension [20], and muscle fiber innervation and size [26, 27]. In addition, we assayed blood serum and muscle IGF-I, and blood serum IGFBPs according to published procedures [29]. Daily treatments of IGF-I (0.02 mg/kg) or GAGs (1 mg/kg) began 24 h after nerve lesioning and terminated the day before animal killing.

The composition of GAGs preparation was as follows: 19.5% slow-moving heparin, 44.9% fast-moving heparin, 28.8% dermatan sulfate, 6.7% chondroitin sulfate A and C. This heparin-enriched preparation has one-fourth the anticoagulant activity of heparin as assessed by APTT (activated pro-thrombin time) evaluation, but it is endowed with similar neuritogenetic and neuroprotective activities [18-20].

Control animals were treated with isovolumetric amounts of saline vehicle. Data are mean ± SDM of at least 6 specimens unless otherwise specified. Statistical differences among experimental groups were evaluated by the Dunnett's *t* test for multiple comparisons, preceded by ANOVA. Statistical significance was accepted at the $P < 0.05$ level. The experimental protocols, approved by the Review Committee of our department, met national guidelines involving laboratory animals, in accordance with the European Communities Council Directive of November 1986 (86/609/EEC).

Results

Grip strength was progressively lossed and gradually declined to low functional levels in vehicle-treated *wobbler* mice. However, both IGF-I and GAGs significantly counteracted this trend. Three weeks after diagnosis, grip strength in vehicle-treated *wobbler* mice was about 50% of initial values, while in drug-treated animals it was around 85% (Fig. 1). The beneficial effects of IGF-I and GAGs were also observed in other behavioral tests such as holding time and running time. Holding time was markedly reduced in vehicle-treated mice, while it was greatly prolonged by either treatment (Fig. 2). Also, the running time of *wobbler* mice was slower than that of heterozygotes and was significantly improved by both drug treatments (Fig. 3). Thus, all three behavioral parameters were significantly improved by administration of IGF-I or GAGs. These data were corroborated by histometric evaluation of biceps muscle fiber size. *Wobbler* mice muscle fibers were smaller on average than controls, and the distribution of sizes was skewed to smaller values (Fig. 4). IGF-I or GAGs administration counteracted the reduced muscle growth, causing fiber size distribution to remain normal. IGF-I and GAGs treatments also affected biceps muscle innervation significantly as shown by combined AChE-silver staining. The innervation pattern was greatly altered by disease: muscle fibers were poorly innervated and sprouting was triggered from the terminal and pre-terminal portions of still healthy axons. Biceps muscle sprouting in vehicle-treated *wobbler* mice was found in 29% (141/486) of the monitored end-plates, while in IGF-I- and GAGs-treated mice the extent of sprouting increased to 43.6% (219/502) and 41.7% (206/494), respectively [25]. However, no effects on *wobbler* mice growth and survival were observed at this stage of the disease. The number of surviving triceps motor neurons in the *wobbler* mouse declined gradually, so that 9 weeks after birth there were around 50 motoneurons in homozygotes compared to over 270 in heterozygotes. Treatment with IGF-I or GAGs doubled the number of surviving motor neurons.

Evaluation of EDL muscle isometric tension in the *Mnd* mouse, 10 months

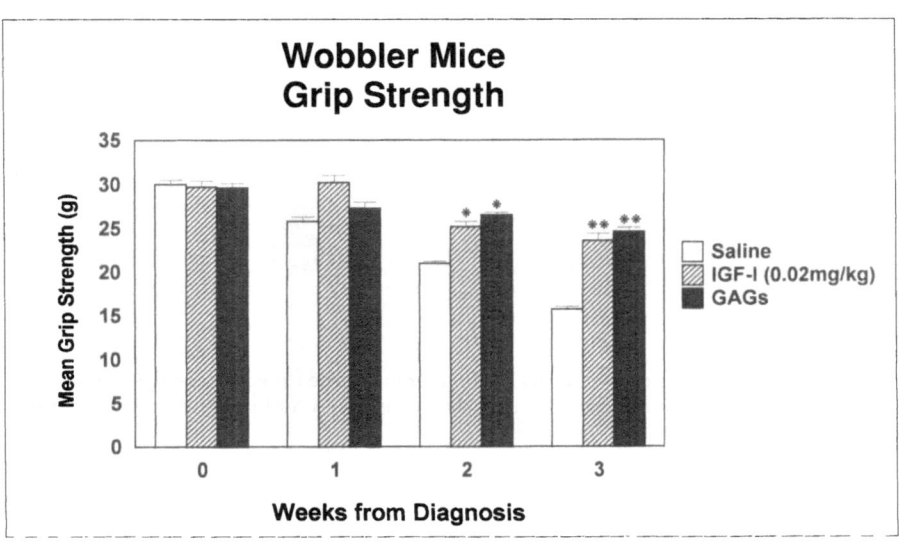

Fig. 1. The progressive decline in *wobbler* mice grip strength is counteracted by IGF-I and glycosaminoglycans (GAGs) treatment. *, P < 0.05; **, P < 0.01

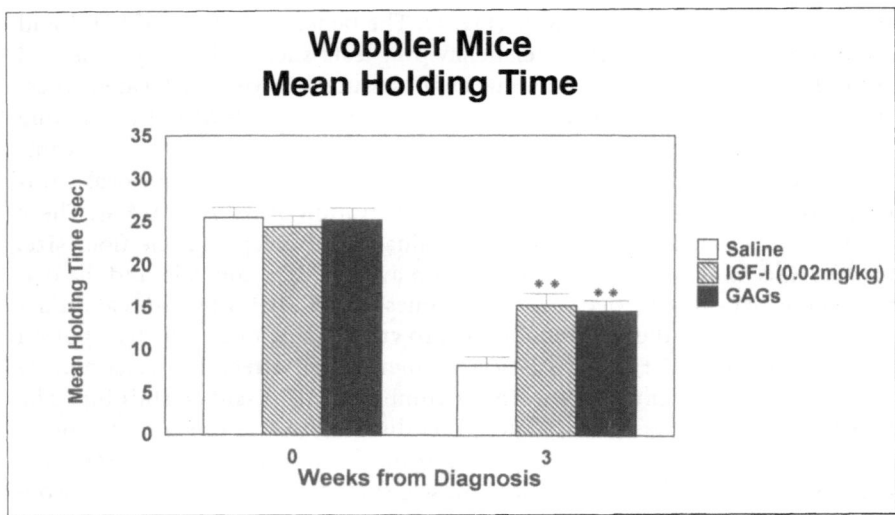

Fig. 2. Holding time is drastically reduced within 3 weeks of diagnosis in *wobbler* mice. IGF-I and GAGs treatments partially counteract the reduction. **, $P < 0.01$

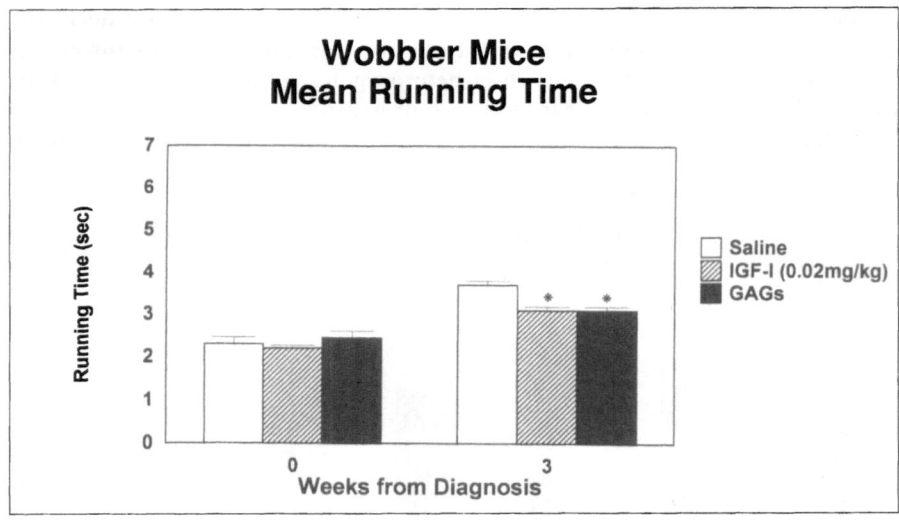

Fig. 3. Running speed is greatly reduced in *wobbler* mice. The time necessary to run a 10 cm stretch is almost doubled at 3 weeks after diagnosis. IGF-I and GAGs treatments significantly reduce the impairment. *, $P < 0.05$

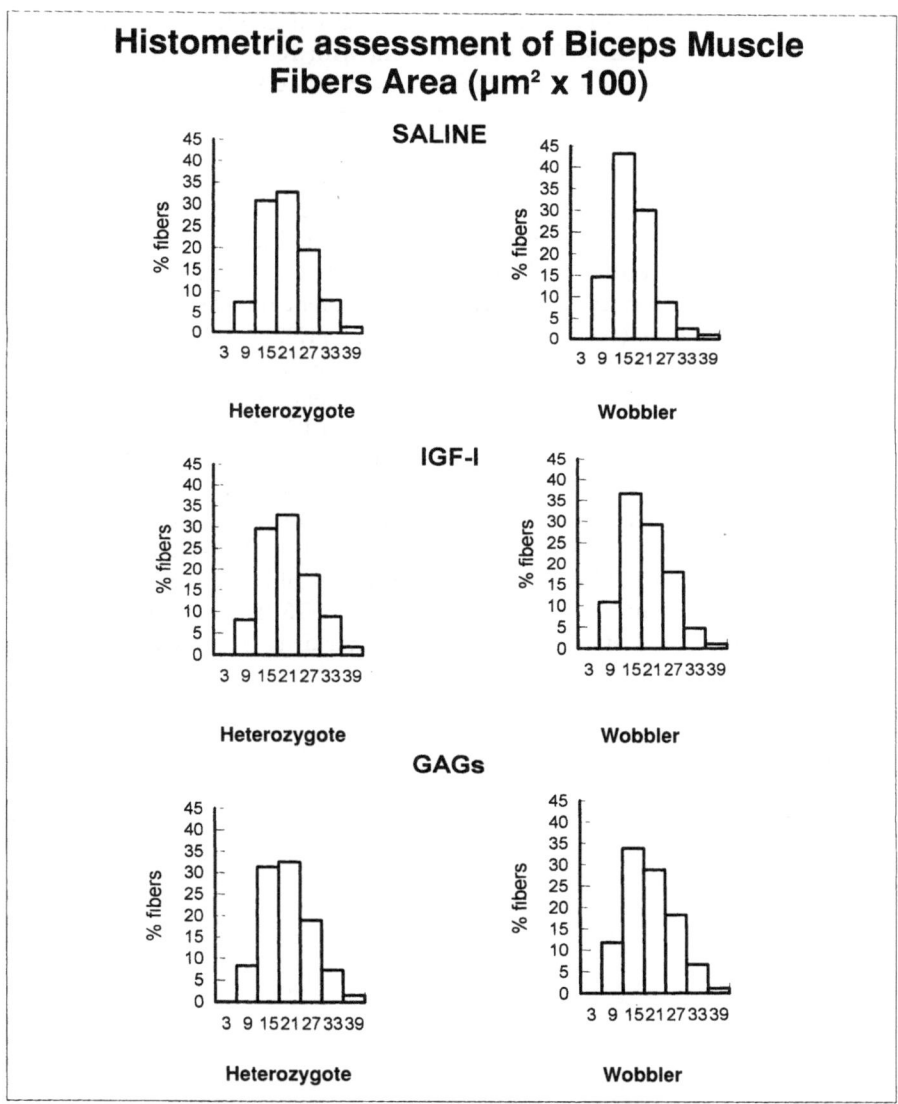

Fig. 4. Muscle fiber size distribution in heterozygotic and homozygotic *wobbler* mice treated with saline, IGF-I, or GAGs. Both treatments significantly reduced the proportion of small fibers (900, 1500 μm²) and augmented that of larger ones (2770, 3300 μm²)

after birth, revealed that high frequency stimulation of the sciatic nerve was unable to trigger EDL muscle tetanus and that the isometric tension dropped to 50% of normal values. Muscles dissected from IGF-I- or GAGs-treated *Mnd* mice had no drop in tetanic isometric tension (manuscript in preparation).

Following neonatal sciatic nerve injury, there is poor reinnervation of the EDL muscle and significant muscle fiber atrophy. When muscle reinnervation

was evaluated 18 days after nerve crush (Fig. 5), 62% of muscle fibers were reinnervated in saline-treated rats while treatment with IGF-I or GAGs increased
the proportion of reinnervated muscle fibers to 75% and 92%, respectively [29].
The distribution of reinnervated EDL muscle fiber areas of saline-treated rats
was skewed to smaller values indicating a prevalence of small, atrophic fibers
(Fig. 6); however, treatments with either IGF-I or GAGs greatly improved the
fiber morphometry resulting in an almost normal size distribution. The effect
was particularly relevant in the group of animals treated with GAGs.

Administration of either IGF-I or GAGs doubled IGF-I mRNA content in
denervated-reinnervated EDL muscle. IGF-I treatment increased IGF-I mRNA
levels from 8.01 ± 0.61 (contralateral muscle) to 11.32 ± 1.01 ng/mg protein
(denervated), while GAGs treatment caused an increase from 7.30 ± 0.62 (contralateral muscle) to 16.21 ± 1.36 ng/mg protein (denervated) in EDL muscles.
In saline-treated rats, there were no differences in IGF-I levels between contralateral and denervated EDL muscles. Both treatments increased IGF-I protein levels 80% in plasma. There was a concomitant increase in blood levels of
IGFBPs (Fig. 7). GAGs treatment induced an almost two-fold increase in IGFBP-
3 levels, without having significant effects on IGFBP-1. IGF-I treatment was
more robust, inducing IGFBP-3 by more than three-fold and IGFBP-1 by one-
fold. Neither treatment altered serum levels of IGFBP-4. These data were
obtained 24 h after the last administration of either drug. Six weeks after nerve

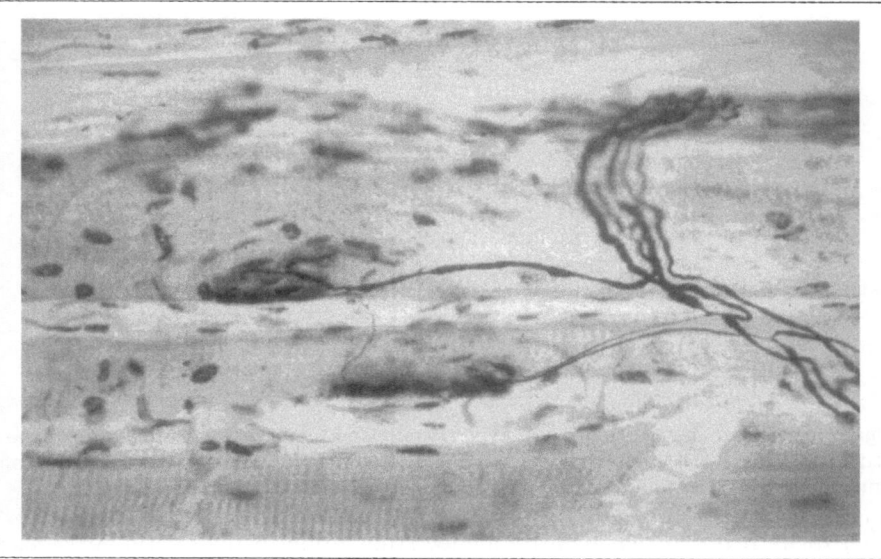

Fig. 5. Silver impregnation and acetylcholinesterase staining of EDL muscle of 21-day-old
rats. Two reinnervated EDL neuromuscular junctions (18 days after nerve lesioning) from
a rat treated with GAGs; one end-plate is reinnervated by two sprouts originated from a
node of Ranvier and by one from the preterminal portion of the other innervating axon

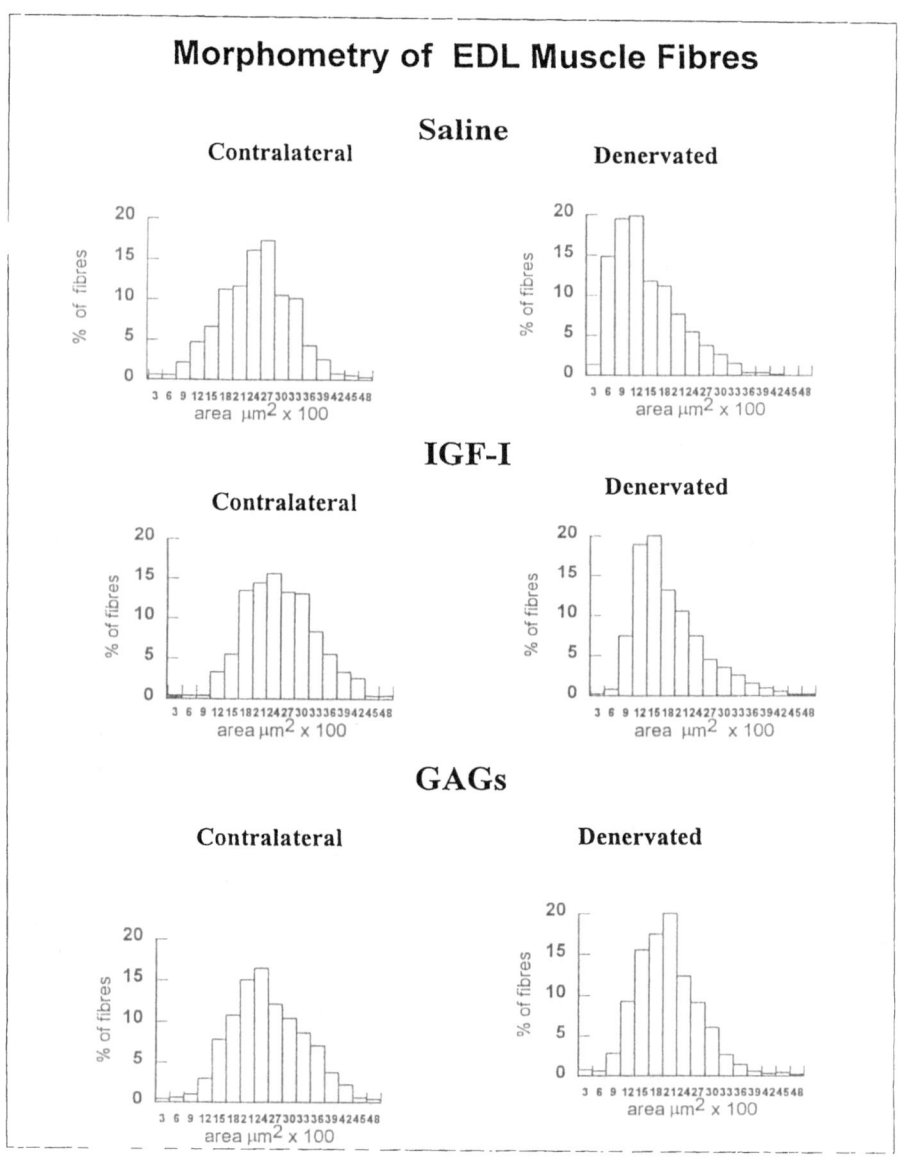

Fig. 6. Muscle fiber size distribution in contralateral and reinnervated EDL muscles 18 days after nerve lesioning. In the reinnervated muscles from saline-treated rats the size distribution is skewed to smaller values with a large number of atrophic fibers; IGF-I and GAGs treatments shift the distribution to the greater values

axotomy, about 70% of all EDL motor neurons were lost; with IGF-I or GAGs treatment, motor neuron death was only about 50%.

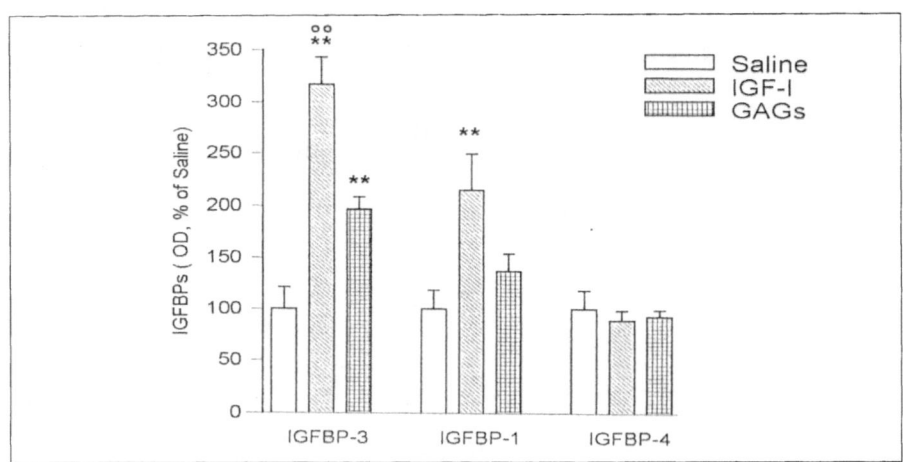

Fig. 7. Plasma levels of insulin-like growth factor binding proteins (IGFBPs) 1, 3, and 4. Following neonatal sciatic nerve injury, rats were treated with IGF-I, GAGs, or saline vehicle. **, $P < 0.01$; *, $P < 0.05$ (IGF-I- or GAGs-treated vs. saline-treated), °°, $P < 0.01$ (IGF-I-treated vs. GAGs-treated)

Discussion

We evaluated the effects of IGF-I treatment on nerve-muscle changes in three different models of motor neuron disease. In addition, we analyzed the novel, non-anticoagulating action of GAGs, recently identified in our laboratory [18-20]. Both IGF-I and GAGs treatments ameliorated muscle reinnervation and function, and promoted motor neuron survival in laboratory models of motoneuron disease.

Diffusible factors must cross the basal lamina before reaching cell surface receptors; thus, binding to specific receptors may be preceded by intermediate binding to extracellular matrix components such as GAGs. For instance, cell-surface, heparin-like molecules bind basic fibroblast growth factor and act as a reservoir, changing its half-life and increasing the cellular response [30]. A similar regulatory process may also occur for IGF-I since heparin, dermatan sulfate and heparan sulfate interact with IGFBPs and reduce IGFBP binding affinity to IGF-I [22, 31]; this would increase availability of IGF-I to its receptor. In addition GAGs affect IGFBP-5 degradation and regulate the interaction of IGFBP-3 with the extracellular matrix [21, 31]. Our data indicate that GAGs increased IGF-I levels in blood and denervated muscles by two mechanisms: a direct promotion of synthesis, as suggested by the higher mRNA levels, and an enhanced rate of IGF-I displacement from the IGFBPs. Both conditions would augment IGF-I availability to its receptor. These studies suggest that GAGs' neuroregenerative and neuroprotective effects are mediated by IGF-I. This view is supported by the finding that IGF-I and GAGs had similar effects in promoting reinnervation of EDL muscle and survival of motor neurons after neonatal sciatic nerve axotomy. Similarly, GAGs and IGF-I had comparable effects in counteracting progressive forelimb muscle weakness and atrophy, and reducing triceps motor neuron loss in the *wobbler* mouse. We previously reported that, following sciatic nerve resection, GAGs administration prevented intraspinal loss of neuropeptides, increased nerve neurotrophin mRNA expression [19], and promoted nerve regeneration and muscle reinnervation after crush lesions [20]. Furthermore, in vitro studies showed that GAGs supplemented to culture medium stimulated neuritogenesis and reduced the requirement for NGF in PC12 differentiation [18].

Low doses of IGF-I promoted nerve regeneration and muscle reinnervation following neonatal nerve injury, prevented nerve-muscle dysfunction in the *Mnd* mouse, and counteracted forelimb muscle atrophy and dysfunction in the *wobbler* mouse. Interestingly, IGF-I administration triggered IGF-I biosynthesis in the denervated muscles. Low doses of GAGs similarly improved nerve muscle repair following neonatal nerve injury and reduced *wobbler* mice impairment, an effect apparently mediated by enhanced IGF-I levels. The two treatments differed in the ability to alter serum levels of IGFBPs which increased more after IGF-I administration. The positive effects induced by GAGs might also be due to contributions of other trophic factors that we and others have shown to be affected by GAGs [18, 19, 32-36].

Acknowledgments

The financial support of Telethon-Italy (grant 671) is gratefully acknowledged. We also thank Pharmacia AB (Stockholm, Sweden) for the supply of IGF-I.

References

1. Gorio A (1993) Neuroregeneration. Raven Press, New York
2. Ramon y Cajal S (1928) Degeneration and regeneration of the nervous system, vol 2. Murray, London
3. Tello JF (1907) Dégéneration et régéneration des plaques motrices. Trav Lab Rech Biol Univ Madrid V:117-149
4. Hamburgher V (1958) Regression versus peripheral control of differentiation in motor hypoplasia. Am J Anat 102:365-409
5. Levi Montalcini R, Hamburgher V (1951) Selective growth-stimulating effects of mouse sarcoma on the sensory and sympathetic nervous system of the chick embryo. J Exp Zool 116:321-361
6. Cohen S, Levi Montalcini R (1956) A nerve growth stimulating factor isolated from snake venom. Proc Natl Acad Sci USA 42:571-574
7. Cohen S (1960) Purification and metabolic effects of a nerve growth-promoting protein from the mouse salivary gland and its neurocytotoxic antiserum. Proc Natl Acad Sci USA 46:302-311
8. Daughaday WH, Hall K, Raben MS, Salmon JL, Van den Brand JL, Van Wyk JJ (1972) Somatomedin: a proposed designation for the "sulfation factor". Nature 235: 107

9.   Lund PK, Moates-Staats BM, Hynes MA, Simmons JG, Jansen M, D'Ercole AJ, Van Wyk
     JJ (1986) Somatomedin-C/insulin-like growth factor-II mRNAs in fetal and adult tis-
     sues. J Biol Chem 261:14539-14544
10   Bohannon NJ, Corp ES, Wilcox BJ, Figlewicz DP, Dorsa DM, Baskin DG (1988)
     Localization of binding sites for insulin-like growth factor-I (IGF-I) in the rat brain
     by quantitative autoradiography. Brain Res 444:205-213
11. Smith M, Clemens J, Kerchner GA, Mendelsohn LG (1988) The insulin-like growth
     factor-II (IGF-II) receptor of rat brain: regional distribution visualized by autoradi-
     ography. Brain Res 445:241-246
12. Bothwell M (1982) Insulin and somatomedin MSA promote nerve growth factor-
     independent neurite formation by cultured chick dorsal root ganglionic sensory neu-
     rons. J Neurosci Res 8:225-231
13. Recio-Pinto E, Rechler MM, Ishii DN (1986) Effects of insulin, insulin-like growth fac-
     tor II, and nerve growth factor on neurite formation and survival in cultured sympa-
     thetic and sensory neurons. J Neurosci 6:1211-1219
14. Aizenman Y, De Vellis J (1987) Brain neurons develop in a serum and glial free envi-
     ronment: effects of transferrin, insulin, insulin-like growth factor-I and thyroid hor-
     mone on neuronal survival, growth and differentiation. Brain Res 406:32-42
15. Caroni P, Grandes P (1990) Nerve sprouting in innervated adult skeletal muscle
     induced by exposure to elevated levels of insulin-like growth factors. J Cell Biol
     110:1307-1317
16. Kanje M, Skottner A, Sjoberg J, Lundborg G (1989) Insulin-like growth factor-I (IGF-
     I) stimulates regeneration of the rat sciatic nerve. Brain Res 486:396-398
17. Hantai D, Akaaboune M, Lagord C, Murawsky M, Houenou LJ, Festoff BW, Vaught JL,
     Rieger F, Blondet B (1995) Beneficial effects of insulin-like growth factor-I on wob-
     bler mouse motoneuron disease. J Neurol Sci 129 [Suppl]:122-126
18. Lesma E, Di Giulio AM, Ferro L, Prino G, Gorio A (1996) Glycosaminoglycans in nerve
     injury: I. Low doses of glycosaminoglycans promote neurite formation. J Neurosci Res
     46:565-571
19. Gorio A, Vergani L, Ferro L, Prino G, Di Giulio AM (1996) Glycosaminoglycans in
     nerve injury: II. Effects on transganglionic degeneration and on the expression of
     neurotrophic factors. J Neurosci Res 46:572-580
20. Gorio A, Lesma E, Vergani L, Di Giulio AM (1997) Glycosaminoglycans promote
     nerve regeneration and muscle reinnervation. Eur J Neurosci (in press)
21. Arai T, Arai A, Busby WH Jr, Clemmons DR (1994) Glycosaminoglycans inhibit
     degradation of insulin-like growth factor-binding protein-5. Endocrinology 135:
     2358-2363
22. Arai T, Parker A, Busby WH Jr, Clemmons DR (1994) Heparin, heparan sulfate, and
     dermatan sulfate regulate formation of the insulin-like growth factor-I and insulin-
     like growth factor-binding protein complexes. J Biol Chem 269:20388-20393
23. Price DL, Cleveland DW, Koliatos VE (1994) Motor neuron disease and animal mod-
     els. Neurobiol Disease 1:3-11
24. Mitsumoto H, Ikeda K, Holmlund T, Greene T, Cedarbaum JM, Wong V, Lindsay RM
     (1994) The effects of ciliary neurotrophic factor on motor dysfunction in wobbler
     mouse motor neuron disease. Ann Neurol 36:142-148
25. Vergani L, Finco C, Di Giulio AM, Muller EE, Gorio A (1997) Effects of low doses of
     glycosaminoglycans and insulin-like growth factor-I on motor neuron disease in
     wobbler mouse. Neurosci Lett (in press)
26. Gorio A, Carmignoto G, Finesso M, Polato P, Nunzi MG (1983) Muscle reinnervation,
     II. Sprouting, synapse formation and repression. Neuroscience 8:403-416

27. Gorio A, Marini P, Zanoni R (1983) Muscle reinnervation, III. Motoneuron sprouting capacity, enhancement by exogenous gangliosides. Neuroscience 8:417-429

28. Messer A, Plummer J, Maskin P, Coffin JM, Frankel WN (1992) Mapping of the motor neuron degeneration *Mnd* gene, a mouse model of amyotrophic lateral sclerosis (ALS). Genomics 18:797-802

29. Gorio A, Vergani L, De Tollis A, Di Giulio AM, Torsello A, Cattaneo L, Müller EE (1997) Muscle reinnervation following neonatal nerve crush. Interactive effects of glycosaminoglycans and insulin-like growth factor-I. Neuroscience (in press)

30. Moscatelli D (1988) Metabolism of receptor-bound and matrix-bound basic fibroblast growth factor by bovine capillary endothelial cells. J Cell Biol 107:753-759

31. Zapf J (1995) Physiological role of the insulin-like growth factor binding proteins. Eur J Endocrinol 132:645-654

32. Li Y, Milner PG, Chauhan K, Watson MA, Hoffman RM, Kodner CM, Milbrandt J, Deuel TF (1990) Cloning and expression of a developmentally regulated protein that induces mitogenic and neurite outgrowth activity. Science 250:1690-1694

33. Merenmies J, Rauvala H (1990) Molecular cloning of the 18 kDa growth-associated protein of developing brain. J Biol Chem 265:16721-16724

34. Serafini T, Kennedy TE, Galko MJ, Mirzayan C, Jessel TM, Tessier-Lavigne M (1994) The netrins define a family of axon outgrowth-promoting proteins homologous to *C. elegans* Unc-6. Cell 78:409-424

35. Tsutsui J, Uehara K, Kadomatsu K, Matsubara S, Muramatsu T (1991) A new family of heparin-binding factors: strong conservation of midkine (MK) sequences between the human and the mouse. Biochem Biophys Res Commun 176:792-797

36. Yamaguchi Y (1993) Proteoglycan-growth factor interaction. Trends Glycosci Glycotechnol 5:428-437

The Potential of IGF-I as a Neuronal Rescue Agent

P. D. Gluckman[1], C. E. Williams[1], J. Guan[1], A. Scheepens[1], R. Zhang[1], V. Russo[2], G. Werther[2]

Introduction

Acute brain injury leads to neuronal and glial death in two phases occurring during and immediately after the insult (assuming the insult is reversed), termed primary neuronal death, and that occurring some hours to days after the injury, termed delayed cell death [1]. The mechanisms contributing to primary cell loss include glutamate toxicity, intracellular calcium accumulation, free radical formation, membrane lipid peroxidation, cytotoxic edema and cell lysis. Programmed cell death (apoptosis) is the most important factor contributing to delayed cell death although the cytotoxic consequences of microglial activation and glutamate toxicity associated with postasphyxial seizures also play a role.

Neuroprotective strategies can address either primary or delayed cell death. Therapies besed on calcium channel antagonists, free radical scavengers or membrane-stabilizing agents which interfere with the processes of primary cell death are most effective when given prior to the insult; this approach is termed neuroprophylaxis. Therapies administered *after* the insult, termed neuronal rescue therapies, are designed to interfere with the processes leading to delayed cell death. Their therapeutic potential is obvious. Delayed cell death plays a major role in perinatal encephalopathy [2], in the development of the penumbra associated with ischemic stroke and in other acute encephalopathies associated with asphyxia, ischemia or trauma. Since patients generally present after injury, then the appropriate strategy is neuronal rescue and the most important biological mechanisms to interrupt are the apoptotic cascade and glutamate toxicity. Apoptosis also plays a major role in a number of neurodegenerative diseases including multiple sclerosis and Huntington's and Alzheimer's diseases [3]. Neuronal rescue agents that interfere with acute apoptosis likely will have roles which extend to the treatment of chronic neurological disease.

[1]Research Centre for Developmental Medicine and Biology, University of Auckland, Private Bag 92019, Auckland, New Zealand and [2]Department of Paediatrics, Royal Childrens Hospital, Melbourne, Australia

Endogenous Neuroprotective Agents

The brain itself attempts to limit injury after an acute insult. The primary processes used include an acute response [4], the release of inhibitory neuromodulators such as γ-aminobutyric acid (GABA) and adenosine, and the induction of neurotrophic agents which possibly limit the apoptotic response by providing neurotrophic support. The original evidence that the brain releases endogenous neurotrophins comes from rats subjected to traumatic brain injury where bioassayable neurotrophin activity was released after 3-10 days [5]. The starting point for our observations was to explore which neurotrophins were induced in rat brain after acute hypoxic-ischemic injury. While neutrophins belonging to the nerve growth factor superfamily were not induced (except in response to postasphyxial seizures), there were marked changes in elements of the insulin-like growth factor (IGF) axis. These observations led us to postulate that IGF-I might be an endogenous neuronal rescue agent with potential therapeutic utility.

Induction of the IGF System Following Brain Injury

We developed a model of graded, unilateral hypoxic-ischemic brain injury in the 21-day-old rat by modifying the Levene preparation [6]. We used in situ hybridization, northern analysis and ribonuclease protection assays to quantitate mRNA induction, and immunohistochemistry to identify cell types and evaluate protein induction.

IGF-I

IGF-I mRNA was expressed at basal levels in the normal brain; following injury there was marked induction which was detected after 3 days and was maximal at 5 days [7]. In situ hybridization showed the IGF-I mRNA to be induced throughout the injured cerebrum including the cortex, striatum, thalamus and hippocampus. The cells expressing the message were primarily activated microglia within the damaged region. With milder degrees of injury leading only to selective neuronal loss, the induction of IGF-I mRNA was largely restricted to those microglial cells adjacent to dead neurons. IGF-I mRNA transcription in the brain used primarily start site 3 in exon 1 of the IGF-I gene, suggesting growth hormone-independent expression (Butler and Gluckman, unpublished results). Immunohistochemistry showed the increased IGF-I protein to be associated with activated microglia plus reactive astrocytes, both proximal and distal to the site of damage.

IGF-II

Constitutive IGF-II expression in the brain was largely restricted to the choroid plexus and the meninges. Brain injury induced IGF-II mRNA to detectable levels after 6 days and to maximal levels at 10 days. Expression was limited to microglial cells and macrophages in the region of cerebral infarction.

Immunohistochemistry showed IGF-II protein to be largely associated with these cells and with reactive, dividing astrocytes on the periphery of the infarct, suggesting a possible role in wound repair [8].

IGF Binding Proteins

IGF binding protein (IGFBP)-2 was found to be constitutively expressed by the choroid plexus; high levels were found in the cerebral spinal fluid (CSF). After injury, IGFBP-2 mRNA was induced in reactive astrocytes, peaking at 3-5 days [9]. The IGFBP-2 protein was localized to neurons, and may therefore be involved in targeting IGF to neurons. Similarly, IGFBP-3 was induced by 3 days after injury [7] and was expressed in these regions by activated microglia. IGFBP-5 was also induced after injury in the subependymal layer and thalamus [10]; some expression was found in neurons. Together, these IGFBPs may target the actions of IGF to specific cells after injury.

There are few studies investigating the roles of IGFs in chronic neurodegenerative disease in vivo. In vitro studies suggest that IGF-I may have unique trophic properties to rescue neurons from amyloid-related toxicity. This effect probably occurs via the IGF-I receptor [11]. We evaluated the expression of IGF-I in brains from patients who suffered from Alzheimer's disease using immunohistochemistry. We observed an induction in reactive astrocytes in regions around the plaques, suggesting a possible role for IGF-I in these lesions [12].

IGF-I as a Neuronal Rescue Agent

Initial studies were performed in the adult rat with unilateral hypoxic-ischemic injury. We used a moderately severe insult (10 min of inhalational asphyxia following ligation of the right carotid artery) which led to infarction in the cerebral cortex and striatum, and to widespread neuronal loss throughout the cerebrum including the hippocampus and thalamus. We evaluated the neuropathological outcome 3-5 days later. A single dose of recombinant human IGF-I (rhIGF-I) administered into the lateral cerebral ventricle 2 h after injury led to a reduction in the incidence of cortical infarction in a dose-dependent manner over the range 5-50 µg/rat. There was a dose-dependent reduction in neuronal loss in all regions-the most marked protective effects were in the thalamus, dentate gyrus and striatum. Administration of rhIGF-I reduced both infarction (regions where both neurons and glia were lost) and selective neuronal loss, suggesting that IGF-I acts on processes common to both necrosis and apoptosis. Neurobehavioural tests such as the sticky patch test of somatosensory function demonstrated that IGF-I therapy gave significant functional improvement.

IGF-I therapy was not effective if given 30 min prior to the injury; this result implies that IGF-I is not effective as a neuronal rescue agent. In pilot studies we have shown IGF-I to be effective when administered as late as 6 h after injury. In the infant (21 day) rat, however, we demonstrated a neuronal rescue action for IGF-I, with differences in the effective dose and distribution of protection. Widespread protection was seen in all regions at high doses of IGF-I following 60 min hypoxic-ischemic injury. Similar trends following milder, 15 min injuries led to selective neuronal loss in most regions apart from in the cortex.

We extended these studies to a paradigm of global cerebral ischemia using the late gestation, fetal sheep preparation [13]. The fetal sheep brain injury paradigm has the advantage that injury is induced in the absence of confounders such as anesthetics, and the intrauterine environment provides effective post-asphyxia support. Sheep brains have relatively precocious development and at this age are almost fully mature. The insult used was 30 min of total cerebral ischemia in late gestation. IGF-I was administered 2 h after injury [14] via an indwelling, lateral, cerebral ventricular catheter. IGF-I was dramatically neuroprotective as evaluated by histopathological analysis 3 days later. The protective effect was evident in the reduced incidence of postasphyxial seizures, reduced magnitude of the secondary rise in cortical impedance, and reduced loss of EEG intensity at 5 days. The distribution of protection was relatively global; both infarction and selective neuronal loss were reduced. The protection was relatively less in the cortex, possibly because this region suffered greater primary neuronal loss in the paradigm used. The most effective dose was 1 µg/fetal sheep (weight 2.5 kg). Doses as low as 100 ng were neuroprotective while doses of 10 µg were not effective. It is not clear why higher doses were not protective-one possibility is that it is due to enhancing metabolic requirements. The range of effective doses of IGF-I was about 10-fold lower than that needed in the rat. Similarly, the doses of rhIGF-I needed to induce anabolism in rats are approximately 10-fold less than those applied in sheep or man. This difference may reflect greater evolutionary diversity of rat IGF-I or differing affinity of rhIGF-I for rat binding proteins.

Action of IGF-I

Studies in rat using telemetry to record brain temperature [15] and in fetal lamb [14] exclude the possibility that IGF-I acts by reducing brain temperature. That IGF-I is active after but not prior to injury suggests an action on delayed cell death. Others have demonstrated that IGF-I inhibits developmental apoptosis in chick embryo fibroblasts. IGF-I appears to inhibit pathological apoptosis in the postasphyxial brain. However, as both infarction and selective neuronal loss are reduced, IGF-I must act at a stage in the death cascade common to necrotic and apoptotic cascades.

In comparison with IGF-I, IGF-II is not neuroprotective when administered at similar doses at the same times. Insulin at comparable doses is not neuroprotective although very high doses have been effective in a forebrain ischemic model [16]; this effect may be due to insulin acting at the type 1 IGF receptor. We also found that des(1-3)IGF-I, which has lower affinity for the IGFBPs, was neuroprotective. These results support our conclusion that IGF-I's neuroprotective effect at physiological concentrations via the type 1 IGF receptor depends on the modifying actions of the IGFBPs [15].

Although in vivo studies indicate that the type 1 IGF receptor has neuronal rescue activity, the precise mechanism of action is unclear. IGF-I was neuroprotective following transient forebrain ischemia in fed [16] but not fasted rats [17], suggesting a possible role in enhancing neural glucose uptake. In vitro [18, 19] IGF-I blocked neuronal apoptosis [20-22]. This effect is mediated (at least in part) by the IGF-I receptor [20], and is associated with an increase in the anti-apoptotic protein Bcl-c(L) [23], but does not involve calcium influx [24].

Transport of IGF-I

We used tritiated IGF-I to evaluate the transport and cellular location of IGF-I administered as a neuronal rescue agent. Autoradiography demonstrated that IGF-I became rapidly concentrated in the region destined to be injured or protected from injury. Maximum concentration occurred with 30 min suggesting an active transport process. Autoradiography demonstrated that IGF-I is transported in the perivascular spaces and along fiber tracts [25]. Transport appeared to be primarily associated with IGFBP-2. IGF-I associated primarily with neuronal cell bodies rather than with other cell types suggesting that IGF-I has a direct neuronal protective action rather than an action mediated through stimulation of glial trophic factor production.

The differential dose response of IGF-I and des(1-3)IGF-I is strongly supportive for a key role of IGFBPs in the neuronal rescue action of IGF-I. The active transport process and the presence of IGF-I in the perivascular space associated with immunoreactive IGFBP-2 further support this postulate. Co-administration of IGF-II (which is not neuroprotective) and IGF-I blocked the neuroprotective action of IGF-I, as well as the uptake of [^{3}H]IGF-I. These results indicate that IGF-II competes with IGF-I for binding sites on IGFBPs and thus reduces the effective concentration of IGF-I. IGF-II administered alone actually increased neuronal loss in some regions of the brain, possibly because IGF-II blocked the localization or action of endogenous IGF-I.

We believe IGFBP-2 to be the key binding protein. The distribution of IGFBP-2 induction upon injury paralleled the sites of neuroprotection. IGFBP-2 mRNA has a biphasic pattern of induction [9] with greater first phase induction in brains with less injury. IGFBP-2 mRNA was expressed in reactive astrocytes juxtaposed to neurons that survived the insult within regions of injury. However IGFBP-3 may also play a role in some regions.

Other Observations with Centrally Administered IGF-I

The administration of IGF-I to asphyxiated rats at effective doses does not appear to be associated with any overt side effects. In the fetal sheep we evaluated cardiovascular status, fetal breathing movements, and blood glucose and lactate, and found no untoward effects at the effective doses. The reduction in postasphyxial seizures was associated with attenuation of the normal post-asphyxial rise in plasma lactate.

Is IGF-I Processed Further?

IGF-I may be proteolytically cleaved in tissues to des(1-3)IGF-I and to an N-terminal tripeptide GPE (glutamate-proline-glycine) [26]. Such proteolytic processing may play part of a mechanism in which IGFBP-2 translocates IGF-I to a target site where protease action reduces the affinity of IGF-I to the binding protein, releasing it to its receptor. Alternatively, IGFBP-2 may be subject to proteolytic processing to reduce its affinity for IGF-I. There is no direct evidence that GPE is produced endogenously. Nevertheless, we evaluated the neuroprotective actions of GPE.

GPE was administered to rats 2 h after hypoxic-ischemic injury via a lateral ventricular cannula. A 3 µg dose (equimolar to the maximally effective dose of IGF-I) was administered. A neuroprotective effect was observed in the cortex, hippocampus and striatum. GPE was protective in CA-1 and CA-2 regions of the hippocampus, regions where IGF-I is not highly neuroprotective and where the concentration of IGF-I receptor is low. Similarly, Gatti et al. (this meeting) have shown GPE to be neuroprotective in rat hippocampal organotypic cultures where neuronal toxicity was induced by N-methyl-d-aspartate (NMDA). The neuroprotective effect of GPE has a broad spectrum. We evaluated the effects of GPE on striatal neuronal cells following hypoxic-ischemic injury. GPE largely prevented asphyxia-induced loss of neurons positive for acetylcholinesterase, glutamate-aspartate dehydrogenase and neuronal nitric oxide synthase (nNOS).

The peptide sequence of GPE suggests that it is an antagonist of the NMDA subtype of glutamate receptor. Such an action has been suggested by the effect of GPE on gonadotrophin control in the hypothalamus [27]. However, when we compared GPE to the NMDA receptor antagonist MK801, GPE was protective at times when MK801 was no longer protective. Furthermore, GPE did not displace various ligands for the NMDA and other glutamate receptors in binding studies. We evaluated the binding of GPE to rat and human brain tissue using autoradiography. GPE binding was greatest in the hippocampus and piriform cortex; however, the distribution of binding sites was not compatible with glutamate receptors. These observations suggest that GPE has neuroprotective action independent of the glutamate receptor. If GPE is actually produced endogenously, then IGF-I may have two modes of action-one via the IGF-I receptor and one through production of GPE.

Other Neuroprotective Growth Factors

Other growth factors such as basic fibroblast growth factor (bFGF) may be neuroprotective. However, the action of bFGF appears indirect: antisera to IGF-I blocked some of the neuroprotective actions of bFGF. Transforming growth factor beta (TGFβ) also acts as a neuronal rescue agent. Several studies reported interactions between the TGFβ and IGF systems. However, the neuroprotective effects of TGFβ are characterized by a narrow dose-response curve which probably will limit its therapeutic utility [28].

Conclusions

Our studies showed marked changes in the IGF system in response to brain injury with an induction of IGF-I, IGFBP-2 and IGFBP-3 in glial cells in the region of injury, suggesting that the IGF-I system may be an endogenous neuroprotector. Administration of IGF-I 2-6 h after injury reduced secondary neuronal loss, suggesting that IGF-I has therapeutic potential as a neuronal rescue agent. The action of IGF-I appears to involve the IGF-I receptor and possibly the generation of GPE which itself appears to neuroprotective. The neuroprotective effect of IGF-I is observed at low doses without obvious side effects. Studies to date have only used centrally administered IGF-I; it is not known whether peripherally administered IGF-I crosses the blood brain barrier sufficiently to be protective.

In the rat, IGF-I administered by lumbar puncture moved retrogradely to the cerebrum. Indeed the flow of cerebrospinal fluid is not only caudal but is also cranial. Thus, in acute brain injury, IGF-I could be administered by several routes. We are considering therapeutic trials of the effectiveness of IGF-I as a neuroprotective agent in cases of perinatal asphyxia via ventricular administration and in cases of adult acute brain injury via lumbar puncture.

Acknowledgments

We acknowledge the contribution of our colleagues Dr. B Johnston, Mr. E Sirimanne, Dr. L Bennet, Dr. A Gunn and Dr. E Beilharz to this work. Our studies are funded by the Health Research Council of New Zealand and NeuronZ Ltd.

References

1. Gluckman PD, Williams CE (1992) When and why do brain cells die? Dev Med Child Neurol 34:1010-1014
2. Roth SC, Edwards AD, Cady EB, Delpy DT, Wyatt JS, Azzopardi D, Baudin J, Townsend J,

Stewart AL, Reynolds EO (1992) Relation between cerebral oxidative metabolism following birth asphyxia, and neurodevelopmental outcome and brain growth at one year. Dev Med Child Neurol 34:285-295

3. Dragunow M, Faull RL, Lawlor P, Beilharz EJ, Singleton K, Walker EB, Mee EW (1995) In situ evidence for DNA fragmentation in Huntington's disease striatum and Alzheimer's disease temporal lobes. Neuroreport 6:1053-1057

4. Tan WKM, Williams CE, During MJ, Mallard CE, Gunning MI, Gunn AJ, Gluckman PD (1996) Accumulation of cytotoxins during the development of seizures and edema after hypoxic-ischemic injury in late gestation fetal sheep. Pediatr Res 39:791-797

5. Nieto-Sampedro M, Lewis ER, Cotman CW, Manthorpe M, Skaper SD, Barbin G, Longo FM, Varon S (1982) Brain injury causes a time-dependent increase in neurotrophic activity at the lesion site. Science 217:860-861

6. Sirimanne ES, Guan J, Williams CE, Gluckman PD (1994) Two models for determining the mechanisms of damage and repair after hypoxic-ischemic injury in the developing rat brain. J Neurosci Methods 55:7-14

7. Gluckman PD, Klempt ND, Guan J, Mallard EC, Sirimanne E, Dragunow M, Klempt M, Singh K, Williams CE, Nikolics K (1992) A role for IGF-I in the rescue of CNS neurons following hypoxic-ischemic injury. Biochem Biophys Res Commun 182:593-599

8. Beilharz EJ, Bassett NS, Sirimanne ES, Williams CE, Gluckman PD (1995) Insulin-like growth factor II is induced during wound repair following hypoxic-ischemic injury in the developing rat brain. Brain Res Mol Brain Res 29:81-91

9. Klempt M, Klempt ND, Gluckman PD (1993) Hypoxia and hypoxia/ischemia affect the expression of insulin-like growth factor binding protein 2 in the developing rat brain. Brain Res 17:347-350

10. Beilharz EJ, Klempt ND, Klempt M, Sirimanne E, Dragunow M, Gluckman PD (1993) Differential expression of insulin-like growth factor binding proteins (IGFBP) 4 and 5 mRNA in the rat brain after transient hypoxic-ischemic injury. Brain Res Mol Brain Res 18:209-215

11. Dore P, Kar S, Quirion R (1997) Insulin-like growth factor I protects and rescues hippocampal neurons against B-amyloid- and human amylin-induced toxicity. Proc Natl Acad Sci USA 94:4772-4777

12. Connor B, Beilharz EJ, Williams CE, Synek B, Gluckman PD, Faull RM, Dragunow M (1997) Insulin-like growth factor 1 (IGF-I) immunoreactivity in the alzheimers disease temporal cortex and hippocampus. Mol Brain Res (in press)

13. Williams CE, Gunn AJ, Gluckman PD, Synek B (1990) Delayed seizures occurring with hypoxic-ischemic encephalopathy in the fetal sheep. Pediatr Res 27:561-565

14. Johnston BM, Mallard EC, Williams CE, Gluckman PD (1996) Insulin-like growth factor-1 is a potent neuronal rescue agent following hypoxic-ischemic injury in fetal lambs. J Clin Invest 97:300-308

15. Guan J, Williams CE, Skinner SJM, Mallard EC, Gluckman PD (1996) The effects of insulin-like growth factor (IGF)-I, IGF-II, and des-IGF-I on neuronal loss after hypoxic-ischemic brain injury in adult rats evidence for a role for IGF binding proteins. Endocrinology 137:893-898

16. Zhu CZ, Auer RN (1994) Intraventricular administration of insulin and IGF-I in transient forebrain ischemia. J Cereb Blood Flow Metab 14:237-242

17. Zhu CZ, Auer RN (1994) Centrally administered insulin and IGF-I in transient forebrain ischaemia in fasted rats. Neurol Res 16:116-120

18. Zhang Y, Tatsuno T, Carney JM, Mattson MP (1993) Basic FGF, NGF, and IGFs protect hippocampal and cortical neurons against iron-induced degeneration. J Cereb Blood Flow Metab 13:378-388

19. Cheng B, Mattson MP (1992) IGF-I and IGF-II protect cultured hippocampal and septal neurons against calcium-mediated hypoglycemic damage. J Neurosci 12:1558-1566
20. Singleton JR, Randolph AE, Feldman EL (1996) Insulin-like growth factor I receptor prevents apoptosis and enhances neuroblastoma tumorigenesis. Cancer Res 56:4522-4529
21. Neff NT, Prevette D, Houenou LJ, Lewis ME, Glicksman MA, Yin QW, Oppenheim RW (1993) Insulin-like growth factors: putative muscle-derived trophic agents that promote motoneuron survival. J Neurobiol 24:1578-1588
22. Deluca A, Weller M, Fontana A (1996) TGF-beta-induced apoptosis of cerebellar granule neurons is prevented by depolarization. J Neurosci 16:4174-4185
23. Parrizas M, LeRoith D (1997) Insulin-like growth factor-1 inhibition of apoptosis is associated with increased expression of the BCL-X(L) gene product. Endocrinology 138:1355-1358
24. Galli C, Meucci O, Scorziello A, Werge TM, Calissano P, Schettini G (1995) Apoptosis in cerebellar granule cells is blocked by high KCl, forskolin, and IGF-I through distinct mechanisms of action: The involvement of intracellular calcium and RNA synthesis. J Neurosci 15:1172-1179
25. Guan J, Skinner SJM, Beilharz EJ, Hua KM, Hodgkinson S, Gluckman PD, Williams CE (1996) The movement of IGF-I into the brain parenchyma after hypoxic-ischemic injury. Neuroreport 7:632-636
26. Sara VR, Carlsson-Skwirut C, Drakenberg K, Giacobini MB, Håkansson L, Mirmiran M, Nordberg A, Olson L, Reinecke M, Ståhlbom PA, Sandberg Nordqvist AC (1993) The biological role of truncated insulin-like growth factor-1 and the tripeptide GPE in the central nervous system. Ann N Y Acad Sci 692:183-191
27. Bourguignon JP, Gerard A, Alvarez Gonzalez ML, Franchimont P (1993) Acute suppression of gonadotropin-releasing hormone secretion by insulin-like growth factor I and subproducts: an age-dependent endocrine effect. Neuroendocrinology 58:525-530
28. McNeill H, Williams CE, Guan J, Dragunow M, Lawlor P, Sirimanne E, Nikolics K, Gluckman PD (1994) Neuronal rescue with transforming growth factor-beta(1) after hypoxic-ischaemic brain injury. Neuroreport 5:901-904

Neurobiology of rhIGF-I: Rationale for Use in Motor Neuron Disease

J. L. VAUGHT, P. C. CONTRERAS, M. MILLER, N. NEFF

Introduction

Recombinant human insulin-like growth factor I (rhIGF-I) is a 70 aminoacid protein with a molecular weight of approximately 7.6 kilodaltons. It was originally identified and isolated based on endocrine and metabolic similarities it shared with insulin, particularly those related to the control of blood sugar. However, intense research has demonstrated that IGF-I is mechanistically, biochemically, and pharmacologically distinct from insulin.

IGF-I is produced by a wide variety of cell types, and is a normally circulating hormone with prominent neurotrophic activity. IGF-I produced locally is important in the growth, development and maintenance of many organ systems, including the nervous system. Immunohistochemical evidence strongly suggests that under normal conditions, IGF-I is expressed in the nervous system of adult animals in discrete areas including anterior horn motor neurons of the lumbar spinal cord, and spinal and autonomic ganglia [1]. In addition, IGF-I synthesis has been detected in astrocytes, glial cells, and skeletal muscle satellite cells.

The cellular effects of IGF-I are mediated by its binding to the Type I IGF receptor, a tetrameric tyrosine kinase receptor that is distinct from the receptor for insulin and other growth factors (e.g. brain-derived neurotrophic factor [BDNF] and ciliary neurotrophic factor [CTNF]). The Type I IGF receptor is broadly distributed and, importantly, is present in the central and peripheral nervous systems where it is found on motor neuron cell bodies, peripheral nerve endings, and muscle [2-5]. The widespread distribution of IGF and its receptor throughout the central and peripheral nervous systems suggests that IGF-I plays a role in the growth, development and function of nervous system tissue, and is important in the regulation of responses to neuronal injury or degeneration.

As shown in Fig. 1, motor neuron disease affects all levels of the neuromuscular axis. Since the precise etiology of sporadic motor neuron disease is unknown, an agent that is active against only one of these disease components would be unlikely to impact the overall clinical state. Thus, a reasonable therapeutic strategy would be to find an agent which affects each of the components

Cephalon Inc., 145 Brandywine Parkway, West Chester, PA 19380 USA

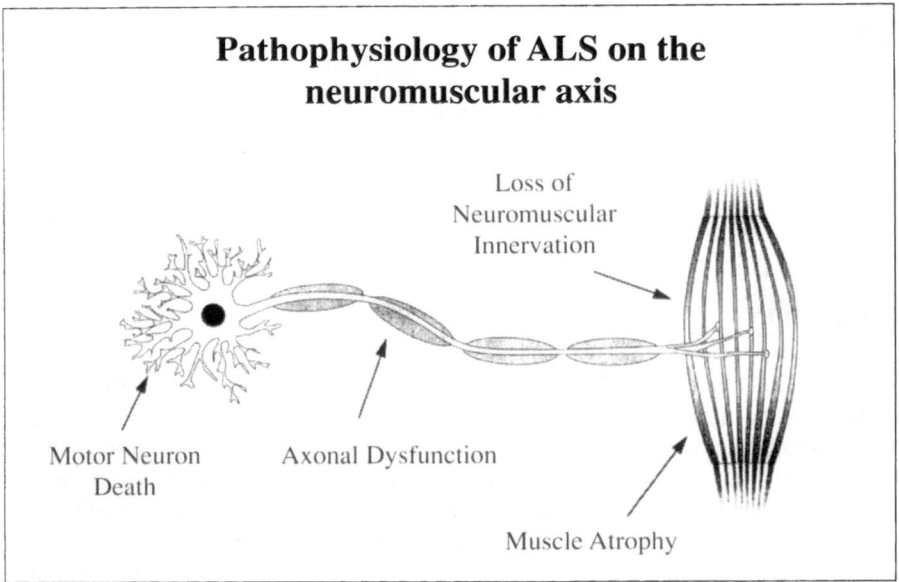

Fig. 1. Pathophysiological consequences of motor neuron disease along the neuromuscular axis include a deficit at the level of the motor neuron, an abnormality in neurofilament function resulting in a dysfunctional axon, denervation at the neuromuscular junction and muscle atrophy. Pharmacological evidence shows IGF-I activity at each of these levels through the promotion of motor neuron survival, enhancement of neuronal sprouting, facilitation of functional recovery following injury, and prevention of decreased muscle mass and strength following denervation

along the neuromuscular axis contributing to disease severity. In this chapter we provide a summary of the evidence demonstrating that IGF-I has prominent restorative actions along the entire neuromuscular axis through the promotion of motor neuron survival, maintenance of muscle innervation, restoration of functional activity, and prevention of decreased muscle mass and strength. Furthermore, we provide evidence that the regenerative activity of IGF-I is a generalized response as it occurs following nerve loss or injury resulting from a variety of insults, including glutamate excitoxicity, a proposed mechanism of motor neuron disease. Finally, we show that subcutaneous administration of rhIGF-I in humans produces serum concentrations comparable to those found to be effective in animal models.

IGF-I Enhances Motor Neuron Survival In Vitro and In Vivo

Neff and colleagues [6] demonstrated that IGF-I promotes survival and neurite outgrowth when added to cultured embryonic day 15 (E15) rat spinal cord neurons enriched for motor neurons. This survival-promoting effect was quantified by measuring choline acetyltransferase (ChAT), a specific biochemical marker for motor neurons. Addition of IGF-I to cultured motor neurons resulted in a concentration-dependent increase in ChAT activity that was approximately 2.5-times greater than that in untreated controls at the highest concentration tested (50 nM). Further, when motor neurons were purified as described by Henderson and colleagues [7], the direct action of IGF-I on motor neuron morphology, phenotype and neurite outgrowth was clearly evident (Fig. 2).

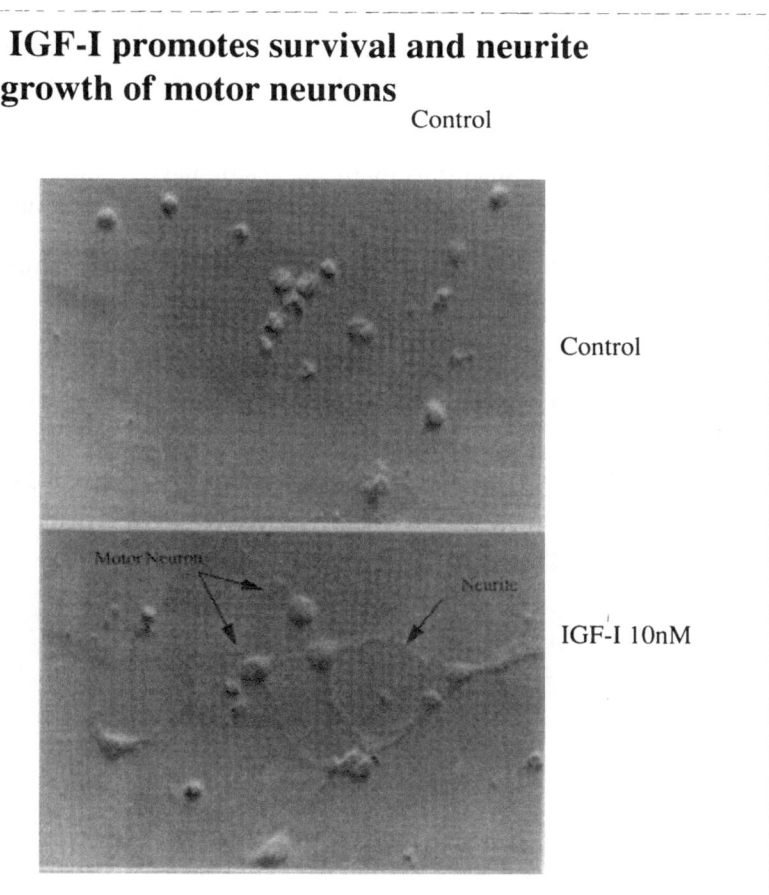

IGF-I promotes survival and neurite outgrowth of motor neurons

Control

Control

IGF-I 10nM

Fig. 2. After two days of culture in a serum- and insulin-free medium, purified embryonic day 15 (E15) rat spinal cord motor neurons begin to die; losing their phenotype and appearing morphologically irregular with no neuritic projection (*right panel*). Addition of IGF-I (10 nM) to the culture (*left panel*) results in a profound survival effect demonstrated by an increase in the number of motor neurons compared to untreated cultures (*below*) and the maintenance of robust cellular morphology and pronounced neuritic extensions (*above*). (From [6])

rhIGF-I also enhanced motor neuron survival in vivo. Within the spinal cord and other regions of the nervous system, many neurons undergo developmentally regulated cell death prior to maturation [8]. This programmed cell death naturally occurs in somatic motor neurons of the developing chick between embryonic days 6 and 10 (E6 and E10). Neff and colleagues [6] demonstrated that administration of rhIGF-I to the chorioallantoic membrane of the chick egg during E6 through E9 promoted survival of spinal motor neurons, with a 25% increase in motor neuron number observed at a 5 µg/egg dose.

Consistent with the above data, rhIGF-I also prevented injury-induced motor neuron death in animals. Hughes et al. [9] demonstrated that application of IGF-I at the nerve stump following facial nerve lesions in newborn rats significantly decreased the loss of facial nerve motor neurons compared to vehicle controls. Li et al. [10] similarly showed that IGF-I administered locally rescued virtually all spinal motoneurons following sciatic nerve axotomy in neonatal mice. Gruner and colleagues [11] studied the effects of IGF-I administered subcutaneously for 7 days following unilateral axotomy of the sciatic nerve in postnatal day 1 mice. As shown in Fig. 3, administration of IGF-I by this clinically

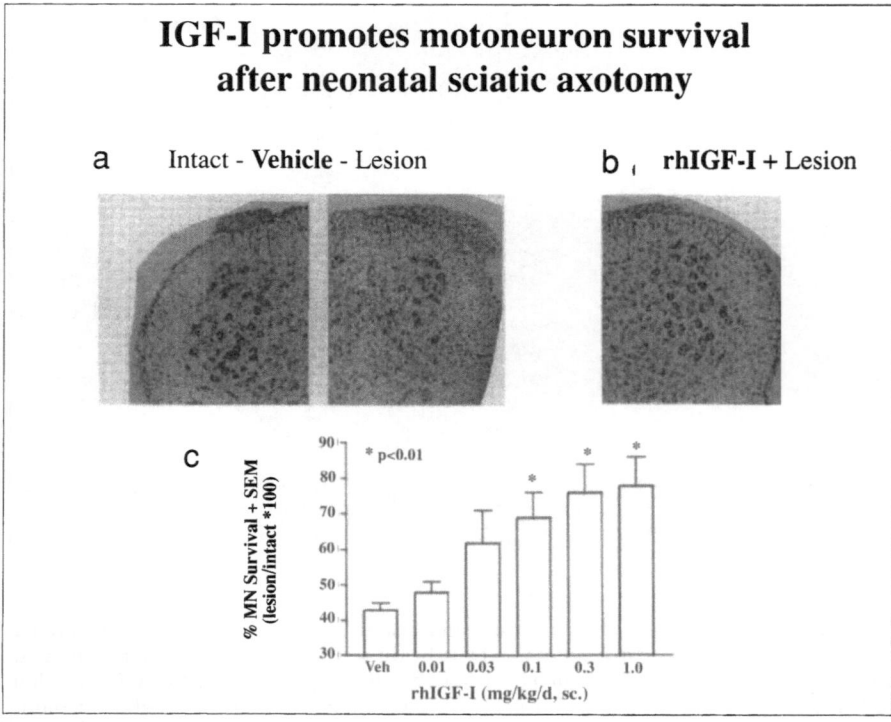

Fig. 3a-c. Unilateral axotomy of the sciatic nerve of neonatal rats on postnatal day 1. **a** Axotomy results in obvious motor neuron loss. **b** Motor neurons are visible on the nonlesioned side. **c** Subcutaneous administraiton of IGF-I promotes the survival of motor neurons. (From [11])

relevant route clearly promoted the survival of sciatic motor neurons destined to die due to axotomy. Similar to the results observed in cell culture, the effects of IGF-I in this model were dose-dependent.

IGF-I Promotes Maintenance of Muscle Innervation and Restores Functional Activity Following Reinnervation

In addition to promoting motor neuron survival, effective treatment of motor neuron disease should involve the maintenance of muscle innervation and subsequent promotion of muscle function. The physiological response of the neuromuscular system to muscle denervation is to reinnervate by an elaboration of sprouts of intramuscular nerves in the vicinity of the denervated muscle. Neuronal sprouts emerging from terminal nerve branches and nodes of Ranvier can reestablish functional contacts with nearby muscle fibers; these new contacts are essential to the restorative process. Patients with motor neuron disease exhibit this compensatory neuronal sprouting in response to neuronal loss [12, 13].

A variety of evidence suggests that IGF-I may be one of the important mediators of the restorative sprouting response to muscle denervation. Caroni and Grandes [14] have shown that subcutaneous administration of IGF-I to the area of the gluteus muscle in rats results in a 10-fold increase of intramuscular nerve sprouts compared to vehicle or unexposed controls. In a later experiment, Caroni [15] induced proliferation of muscle interstitial cells and sprouting of motor neurons in mouse gluteus muscle through subcutaneous administration of botulinum toxin. He then demonstrated that the sprouting effect in botulinum toxin-paralyzed muscle could be completely neutralized by the addition of IGF binding protein 4 (IGFBP-4), a specific IGF-I binding protein which blocks the actions of IGF-I. These data suggest that IGF-I is the key endogenous sprouting factor. Based on these findings, it is likely that administration of exogenous IGF-I could supplement the physiological process that mediates motor neuronal sprouting, thus providing additional rationale for its use in the therapy of motor neuron disease [16].

Although enhancement and maintenance of motor neuron sprouting are desirable therapeutic attributes, to be clinically useful in motor neuron disease they must be associated with recovery of motor function. To examine the functional consequences of the regenerative activity of IGF-I, Contreras and colleagues [17] utilized a model of sciatic nerve injury in which the sciatic nerve of the mouse is gently crushed resulting in a transient loss of function that gradually recovers over the course of 7-21 days. Daily subcutaneous administration of IGF-I (at doses ranging from 0.1 to 30 mg/kg) immediately following injury accelerated recovery of motor function in a dose-dependent manner (Fig. 4). Maximal effects were observed at the 1 mg/kg dose level. The chronology of this response was similar to the motor neuron sprouting response described above, and is therefore consistent with sprouting resulting in the enhanced recovery of motor function.

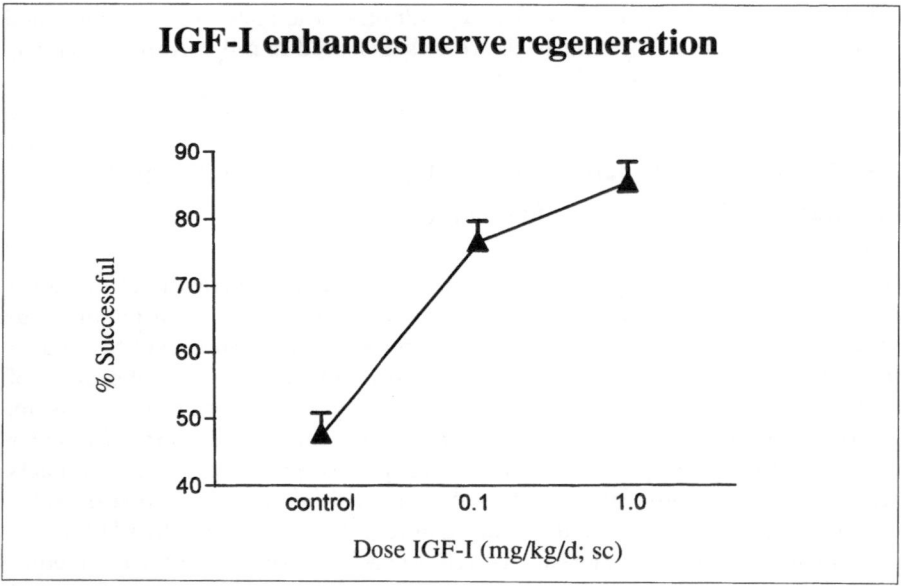

Fig. 4. IGF-I promotes recovery of grip strength following sciatic nerve crush. Each mouse was tested 5 times for the ability to grip an inverted wire screen. By day 12, mice that received no IGF-I succeeded on 46% of their attempts. Subcutaneous administration of IGF-I at dosages of 0.1 and 1.0 mg/kg/d increased the number of successful attempts to 77% and 82%, respectively. (From [17])

IGF-I in a Genetic Model of Motor Neuron Degeneration

With the exception of developmentally regulated cell death in the chick, each of the previously mentioned experiments involved an induced injury rather than a functional deficit caused by an endogenous physiologic process. The *wobbler* mouse provides a genetically defined, naturally occurring model of motor neuron degeneration. Mice bearing this autosomal recessive trait exhibit forelimb muscle dysfunction, weakness and atrophy beginning approximately 3 weeks after birth. Hantai et al. [18] showed that daily subcutaneous administration of IGF-I (1 mg/kg) to *wobbler* mice over a postnatal period of 4-10 weeks results in a statistically significant improvement in grip strength compared to vehicle-treated controls (Fig. 5). In addition to increased functional grip strength, subcutaneous administration of IGF-I slowed the deterioration in muscle fiber diameter, an indication of IGF's ability to slow muscle atrophy in this genetic model of motor neuron disease. Vergani and colleagues [19] recently confirmed and extended these data by demonstrating that the maintenance of grip strength in IGF-I-treated *wobbler* mice (compared to control mice) is correlated with a concomitant reduction in the number of atrophic small fibers [20].

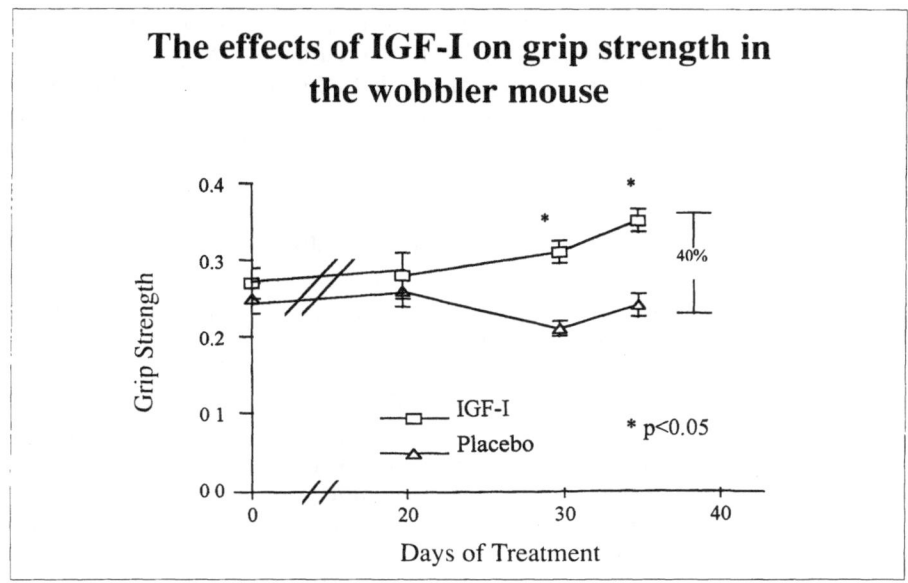

Fig. 5. Subcutaneous administration of IGF-I prevents the deterioration of grip strength in the *wobbler* mouse model of motor neuron disease. Grip strength was quantified by the use of a dynamometer. A decline in the placebo-treated group was observed starting at approximately week 3. Subcutaneous IGF-administration of 1 mg/kg IGF-I significantly improved grip strength compared to placebo. (From [18])

IGF-I in a Model of Glutamate Excitotoxicity

Despite the increased understanding of the areas of the neuromuscular axis affected in motor neuron disease, the specific etiology of the sporadic form of the disease, which constitutes 90% of cases, remains unknown. A possible mechanism suggested by Rothstein and colleagues [21] involves a prolonged elevation of extracellular glutamate, a mediator of excitotoxic neuronal death, in the cerebrospinal fluid. The cause of this elevation of glutamate is thought to be a selective loss from spinal cord glia of the high-affinity glutamate transporter which is responsible for clearing and regulating the levels of glutamate in the synaptic environment. Rothstein and his colleagues [22] have further demonstrated that a knockout of the glutamate transporter gene can induce motor neuron pathology both in vitro and in vivo.

In collaboration with Rothstein, Corse and Kuncl, IGF-I was evaluated in rat spinal cord organotypic cultures where glutamate toxicity was produced slowly over the course of several weeks by pharmacological inhibition of the glutamate transporter, resulting in an elevation of extracellular glutamate [manuscript in preparation]. After 6 weeks of increased extracellular glutamate, histologic evaluation revealed a near complete loss of motor neurons in control cultures. Addition of IGF-I (100 ng/ml) to the culture medium prevented the glutamate-induced loss of neurons. A 3-fold increase in ChAT activity was also observed in the IGF-I-treated culture. Although further understanding of the precise disease mechanisms is needed, these results indicate that IGF-I can attenuate the toxic effects of glutamate, a potentially important pathogenic factor in motor neuron disease.

Comparison of Serum Concentrations in Animals and Humans

For other growth factors, the concentrations observed in preclinical animal models sometimes exceeded those achievable in human dosing. Therefore, we investigated whether the serum concentrations of IGF-I achieved in preclinical animal models were comparable to those which would occur in patients with motor neuron disease who were treated with rhIGF-I. Contreras and colleagues [17] found that the subcutaneous doses of IGF-I which effectively promoted recovery of motor function following sciatic nerve injury in mice also resulted in dose-dependent elevations in serum IGF-I concentrations. We have subsequently found that the maximum serum concentrations achieved in these mice after an optimal dose of rhIGF-I are comparable to those resulting from administration of rhIGF-I at 0.05 mg/kg once or twice daily to humans with motor neuron disease.

Discussion

The data summarized in this chapter represent the neurobiological rationale behind the investigation of the utility of IGF-I in motor neuron disease. We and others have compiled a wealth of evidence indicating that IGF-I promotes the survival of motor neurons, enhances neuronal sprouting, facilitates functional recovery following injury, and decreases the loss of muscle mass and strength following denervation. These actions represent the activity of rhIGF-I at all levels of the neuromuscular axis compromised in motor neuron disease. Furthermore, we have shown that IGF-I is active in a variety of models of nerve loss or injury, including a model of glutamate-induced excitoxicity. Finally, we have shown that subcutaneous administration of rhIGF-I at dosages of 0.05 mg/kg once or twice daily in humans produces serum concentrations comparable to those found to promote functional recovery of injured motoneurons in mice. These findings provide a strong pharmacological rationale for the investigation of the therapeutic utility of IGF-I in patients with motor neuron disease.

Acknowledgements

The authors greatly appreciate the assistance from Linda Hartman, RPh and Watson Laughton, PhD in the preparation of this chapter.

References

1. Hansson H-A, Rozell B, Skottner A (1987) Rapid axoplasmic transport of insulin-like growth factor I in the sciatic nerve of adult rats. Cell Tissue Res 247:214-247
2. Sara VR, Hall K, Von Holtz H, Humbel RE, Sjogren B, Wetterberg L (1982) Evidence of the presence of specific receptors for insulin-like growth factors 1 (IGF-1) and 2 (IGF-2) and insulin throughout the adult human brain. Neurosci Lett 34:38-44
3. Baskin DG, Wilcox BJ, Figlewicz DP, Dorsa DM (1988) Insulin and insulin-like growth factors in the CNS. Trends Neurosci 11:107-111
4. Baron-Van Evercoon B-A, Olichon-Berthe C, Kowalski A, Visciano G, Van Obberghen E (1991) Expression of IGF-I and insulin receptor genes in the rat central nervous system: a developmental, regional, and cellular analysis. J Neurosci Res 28:244-253
5. Kar S, Chabot J-G, Quirion R (1993) Quantitative autoradiographic localisation of [^{125}I]insulin-like growth factor I, [^{125}I]insulin-like growth factor II, and [^{125}I]insulin receptor binding sites in developing and adult rat brain. J Comp Neurol 333:375-397
6. Neff NT, Prevette D, Houenou LJ, et al (1993) Insulin-like growth factors: putative muscle-derived trophic agents that promote motoneuron survival. J Neurobiol 24:1578-1588
7. Henderson CE, Huchet M, Changeux JP (1983) Denervation increases a neurite promoting activity in extracts of skeletal muscle. Nature 302:609-611
8. Oppenheim RW (1991) Cell death during development of the nervous system. Annu Rev Neurosci 14:453-501
9. Hughes RA, Sendtner M, Thoenen H (1993) Members of several gene families influence survival or rat motoneurons in vitro and in vivo. J Neurosci Res 36:663-671
10. Li LX, Oppenheim RW, Lei M, Houenou LJ (1994) Neurotrophic agents prevent motor neuron death following sciatic nerve section in the neonatal mouse. J Neurobiol 25:759-766
11. Gruner JA, Wagner L, Bhat RV, Contreras PC, Miller MS (1997) rhIGF-I promotes motoneuron survival following neonatal sciatic transection. 27th Annual Meeting, Society for Neuroscience, October 25-30, 1997, New Orleans, A248.19
12. Bjornskov EK, Norris FH Jr, Mower-Kuby J (1984) Quantitative axon terminal and end-plate morphology in amyotrophic lateral sclerosis. Arch Neurol 41:527-530
13. Dengler R, Konstanzer A, Kuther G, Hesse S, Wolf W, Struppler A (1990) Amyotrophic lateral sclerosis: Macro-EMG and twitch forces of single motor units. Muscle Nerve 13:545-550
14. Caroni P, Grandes P (1990) Nerve sprouting in innervated adult skeletal muscle induced by exposure to elevated levels of insulin-like growth factors. J Cell Biol 110:1037-1317
15. Caroni P (1993) Activity-sensitive signals by muscle-derived insulin-like growth factors in the developing and regenerating neuromuscular system. Ann N Y Acad Sci 692:209-222
16. Lewis ME, Neff NT, Contreras PC, et al (1993) Insulin-like growth factor-I: potential for treatment of motor neuronal disorders. Exp Neurol 124:73-88
17. Contreras PC, Steffler C, Yu E, Callison K, Stong D, Vaught J (1995) Systemic administration of rhIGF-I enhanced regeneration after sciatic nerve crush in mice. J Pharmacol Exp Therap 274:1443-1499
18. Hantai D, Akaabourne M, Lagord C, et al (1995) Beneficial effects of insulin-like growth factor-I on Wobbler mouse motoneuron disease. J Neurol Sci 129:122-126
19. Vergani L, Finco C, Di Giulio AM, Müller EE, Gorio A (1997) Effects of low doses of glycosaminoglycans and insulin-like growth factor-I on motor neuron disease in wobbler mouse. Neurosci Lett 228:41-44

20. Gorio A, Vergani L, Losa M, Pezzoni G, Calvano L, Finco C, Di Giulio AM, Torsello A, Müller EE (1998) IGF-I and glycosaminoglycans improve peripheral nerve regeneration and motor neuron survival in models of motor neuron disease. In: Müller EE (ed) IGFs in the Nervous System. Springer-Verlag, Berlin Heidelberg New York, pp 84-85
21. Rothstein JD, Martin LJ, Kuncl RW (1992) Decreased glutamate transport by the brain and spinal cord in amyotrophic lateral sclerosis. N Engl J Med 326:1464-1468
22. Rothstein JD, Jin L, Dykes-Hoberg M, Kuncl RW (1993) Chronic inhibition of glutamate uptake produces a model of slow neurotoxicity. Proc Natl Acad Sci USA 90:6591-6595

rhIGF-I for the Treatment of Neuromuscular Disorders

V. Silani[1], A. Brioschi[1], A. Sampietro[1], A. Ciammola[1], A. Pizzuti[1, 2], G. Scarlato[1]

Introduction

Type I insulin-like growth factor-I (IGF-I) receptors are widely distributed throughout the nervous system, suggesting an important role for IGF-I in the growth, development, and maintenance of the central nervous system (CNS). This, in part, has been the stimulus for extensive studies on the actions of IGF-I on muscle and in the CNS. *In vitro*, IGF-I induces differentiation of muscle cells, prevents myoblast apoptosis and promotes survival of several neuronal types. Furthermore, IGF-I has been shown to stimulate *in vitro* the proliferation of neuronal progenitor cells and to increase the survival of both neurons and oligodendrocytes. *In vivo*, IGF-I has profound effects on neuronal and skeletal muscle development including increases in motor neuron sprouting, rate of neuronal recovery after injury, and muscle mass [1]. This pre-clinical evidence suggests that IGF-I may have beneficial effects in pathological conditions characterized by motor neuron loss, denervation, and skeletal muscle atrophy. Recently, the efficacy of recombinant human IGF-I (rhIGF-I) has been studied in patients with amyotrophic lateral sclerosis, post-polio syndrome and myotonic dystrophy. In addition, indirect data from one clinical study suggested that IGF-I may mediate the clinical benefit provided by prednisone in the treatment of Duchenne muscular dystrophy.

Amyotrophic Lateral Sclerosis

Amyotrophic lateral sclerosis (ALS) is a fatal disease involving progressive upper and lower motor neuron deterioration at multiple levels of the neuraxis. While there has been an intensive research effort to elucidate the aetiology of the disease, the underlying cause has remained elusive. For approximately 10% of patients, an autosomal dominant pattern of inheritance has been determined, and, in about one-half of these, a genetic mutation of the superoxide dismutase (SOD) gene has been demonstrated [2]. For the remaining 90% of

[1]The Institute of Neurology, University of Milan Medical School and I.R.C.C.S. Maggiore Hospital, Milan, Italy, [2]C.S.S. Hospital and I.R.C.C.S. San Giovanni Rotondo, Foggia, Italy

patients with so-called sporadic ALS, no genetic predisposition has been identified. Immunologic, neurotoxic, and excitotoxic hypotheses are under active consideration.

The involvement of trophic factors in ALS is one hypothesis on the aetiology of this condition. It has been postulated that motor neuron death in ALS may result from deficient production and/or release of trophic factors by skeletal muscle or other tissues, or from attenuation of the normal action of these factors due to receptor dysfunction, disturbed axonal transport or diminution of soluble factor(s) due to antibody or binding protein effects [3]. If this hypothesis has any validity then, clearly, treatment of ALS with exogenous trophic factors would be justified. Alternatively, given the broad role of IGF-I in the recovery and maintenance of neuronal cells, supraphysiological amounts of trophic factors may assist motor neurons in "managing" damage caused by other pathological processes in ALS. This concept has been the stimulus for pre-clinical and clinical studies in ALS.

Pre-clinical animal data provide strong evidence that rhIGF-I may have a role in the treatment of ALS. Obviously, it is extremely difficult to extrapolate from *in vitro* and *in vivo* animal data to human clinical settings. Kerkhoff et al. [4] studied the distribution of immunoreactive IGF in the neuromuscular system of patients with ALS and in a group of control patients. IGF immunoreactivity was demonstrated in the cell bodies and axons of motor neurons, in astroglia, Schwann cells, and skeletal muscle fibres. There was no difference in the distribution of IGF-I immunoreactivity between samples from control and ALS patients. Thus, ALS does not appear to be associated with a deficiency of IGF-I production. Braunstein and Reviczky [5] showed that serum concentrations of IGF-I in patients with ALS were not significantly different from control values and suggested that binding of antibody to IGF-I was not the cause of motor neuron degeneration. Doré et al. [6] studied the distribution and density of IGF-I receptors in spinal cord samples from ALS patients and controls. The cords from ALS patients showed increased binding of IGF-I in most areas but particularly in the ventral horn and intermediate zone. It is not clear from these data which cell phenotype, i.e. neurone or astrocyte, overexpressed IGF-I receptors. Similar findings have been reported by Adem et al. [7]. Thus, experimental data suggest that ALS patients are "primed" for IGF-I. If the actions of IGF-I in humans are similar to those in experimental animals, then this agent may well have a beneficial effect on ALS.

The clinical applicability of this hypothesis has been explored in two recent, multicentre studies. The first of these studies was conducted in North America while the second was in Europe. In both studies the response to treatment was assessed using functional criteria rather than survival as was used in the studies of the glutamate antagonist riluzole [8, 9]. It was considered at the outset that changes in function would have more relevance to patients and clinicians in this debilitating, rapidly progressive and ultimately fatal illness. The Appel ALS (AALS) rating scale was used to assess disease progression. The total score of the AALS scale is a summation of individual objective and subjective functional measures and has been validated as an accurate index of disease severity [10]. The rate of change of total score correlates well with disease progression and it is a predictor of survival. This scale is reproducible, easy to administer, and uses traditional methods of assessment such as forced vital capacity (FVC), manual muscle testing, and timed walking distances. The test assesses five functional domains using standardized methodology (Table 1). As the disease progresses the AALS score increases. An increment of 20 points is indicative of increasing disability resulting in a major change in patient lifestyle (Table 2).

In the North American study 266 patients with sporadic ALS participated. Patients with AALS scores between 40 and 80 (mild to moderate disease severity) were eligible for randomization if their AALS score had increased by at least 5 points during a 2-3 month screening period. In addition, participating patients were aged 20 years or older and had had symptoms of ALS for fewer than 3 years. The patients were randomized to either placebo, rhIGF-I at 0.05 mg/kg per day (low dose), or rhIGF-I at 0.10 mg/kg per day (high dose). The study in medication was administered subcutaneously under double-blind conditions over 9 months, since the response to therapy may depend upon the status of the patient on entry into the study, patients were stratified according to whether the AALS score was 60 or less, or greater than 60. Following randomization, the functional

Table 1. Appel ALS scale functional domains (from [10])

Functional domain	Tests	Points
Bulbar	Swallowing Speech	6 - 30
Respiratory		6 - 30
Muscle strength	Upper extremity Lower extremity Grip Lateral pinch	6 -36
Muscle function, lower extremity	Standing from chair Standing from supine Walking 20 feet Assistive devices Climb/descend stairs Hips/legs	6 - 35
Muscle function, upper extremity	Dress/feed Wheelchair Arms/shoulders Cutting Pegboard Blocks	6 - 33
Total score		164

Table 2. Lifestyle deterioration on the Appel ALS scale (Adapted from [10])

Function	Appel score		
	52	75	99
Diet	General to soft	Soft	Pudding
Mobility	Possible cane	Walker / occasional wheelchair	Wheelchair most of the time
Independence	Independent	Caretaker assistance	Caretaker provides most of the care

status of the patients was evaluated monthly (AALS). Periodically, other clinical and laboratory observations were made. In order to monitor the impact of the treatment on patient-perceived quality of life, the Sickness Impact Profile (SIP) was administered at baseline and at 3 month intervals. SIP measures 12 health-related quality-of-life categories and was carried out, independently of the clinical evaluations, by trained personnel in telephone interviews with each patient.

As described above, the AALS, in particular the slope of AALS scores with time was the main efficacy measure. Other derivatives of the AALS score were used to assess therapeutic effect as follows:

1. The change in AALS score from baseline to the end of the study
2. The time taken for the AALS score to increase to 115 or greater, or for the FVC to decrease to less than 39% of predicted, at which point the study was terminated
3. The time taken for a 20-point increase in AALS score

Results from this study have been reported [11, 12]. Of the 266 patients enrolled, 141 completed the 9-month study period. Of the 125 patients withdrawn from the study, 67 patients (29 placebo, 23 low dose and 15 high dose) reached the protocol-specified termination criteria (AALS ≥ 115 or FVC < 39% predicted), 26 patients (7 placebo, 11 low dose, and 8 high dose) died during the study, 32 patients withdrew for a variety of other reasons. Analysis of the efficacy data showed that the rate of disease progression, defined by the rate of change of the AALS score, was decreased by administration of rhIGF-I in a dose-related manner. The difference in rates between the high dose rhIGF-I-treated and the placebo groups reached statistical significance ($P = 0.01$). Similarly, the time taken for a 20-point increase in the AALS score was significantly increased ($P = 0.001$) in those patients receiving rhIGF-I at 0.10 mg/kg day.

Further examination of the AALS component scores showed an effect of high dose rhIGF-I on each of the components, with the most consistent effects observed in bulbar function, muscle strength, and muscle function of the arm. The therapeutic effect of rhIGF-I as evaluated by the AALS score was supported by the SIP results, with statistically significant differences being observed in changes in SIP score between those receiving high dose rhIGF-I and the placebo group. Patients with more rapidly progressing disease at the start of the study responded in a more pronounced manner to rhIGF-I than those with more slowly progressing disease. The drug was generally well tolerated and no clinically significant, adverse effects were encountered.

The multinational European study, although broadly similar in design to the North American study, differed in several important respects:

1. Two treatment arms only-placebo or rhIGF-I at 0.10 mg/kg day;
2. The ratio of patients randomized to placebo or rhIGF-I was 1:2;
3. The primary efficacy variable was the change in AALS total score from baseline;
4. Stratification according to initial severity was not carried out.

As a result of the 1:2 randomization, the number of patients in the control group was relatively small, reducing the power of the study to detect a significant treatment effect. Preliminary results from this study have been communicated [13]. Compared with those receiving placebo, patients receiving rhIGF-I had lower AALS scores at the end of the study, although the change from baseline was not significantly different between the groups. Post hoc analysis of the slope of the AALS scores showed a slower rate of progression in the rhIGF-I group compared to the placebo group, although the difference did not reach statistical significance. The data from this study are thus directionally consistent with, but not as robust as, the North American data. The failure to reach statistical significance probably relates to the inadequate power of this study to detect significant changes.

In view of the similarities in study design and data analysis techniques, the data from the placebo and high dose rhIGF-I treated patients in the North American study were combined with the data from the European study in a pooled analysis [14]. This analysis showed that the difference in AALS slopes between the rhIGF-I treatment and placebo groups was -0.8 points/month ($P = 0.04$). Similarly, analysis of the change in AALS scores from baseline demonstrated a difference between the groups in favour of rhIGF-I of -4.6 points ($P = 0.009$). Further examination showed effects on individual components of the AALS score with significant slowing of disease progression for bulbar function ($P = 0.02$), muscle strength ($P = 0.009$), and upper extremity muscle function ($P = 0.02$). Time-to-event analyses were conducted using the Cox proportional hazards model. Over the 9 month treatment period, patients receiving rhIGF-I demonstrated a 40% lower risk of reaching protocol termination criteria and a 26% lower risk of developing a 20-point increase in AALS score compared with those receiving placebo.

The results from these two important studies demonstrate that rhIGF-I administered subcutaneously as a twice daily injection of 0.05 mg/kg slows the rate of progression of ALS. The results are statistically significant in the North American study but not so in the European one probably because of lack of power of the latter study. The attenuation of disease progression is modest but in this rapidly progressive condition in which treatment is started only after destruction of a significant proportion of motor neurons, it may be unrealistic to expect more dramatic effects at this early stage in the development of pharmacological intervention. Furthermore, these modest changes were supported by significant changes in health-related quality of life as measured by SIP.

During the introduction of chemotherapy for the treatment of malignancies, similar reductions in tumour progression were noted. However, developments in oncology, particularly the multi-drug approach to treatment, have lead to significant improvements in responses to some tumours. It is hoped that progression in the medical treatment of ALS will proceed in a similar manner. As a priority, the possibilities of improved therapeutic responses to combinations of drugs such as rhIGF-I and riluzole require evaluation.

Post-Polio Syndrome

The post-polio syndrome (PPS) occurs many years after an episode of paralytic polio. Following a protracted period of neurological and functional stability, which may be as long as 20-30 years, the patient presents with muscular weakness, fatigue, and decreased endurance often accompanied by muscular atrophy. Electrophysiological examination frequently shows evidence of acute denervation superimposed on chronic denervation-reinervation. The pathophysiological basis for the condition has not been resolved. Sharma et al. [15] examined the fatigability of the anterior tibial muscle in patients with PPS using measurements of muscle force, metabolism, membrane function, neuromuscular transmission, excitation-contraction coupling, and central fatigue during intermittent, low intensity, isometric voluntary exercise. They found that maximal voluntary contraction declined significantly more and muscle subsequently recovered significantly less in patients with PPS compared to a group of control patients, confirming greater muscle fatigue in the PPS patients. On the basis of metabolic and other studies, it was suggested that the impairment of muscle function in these patients results from dysfunction in excitation-coupling [15].

Miller et al. [16] argued that the pharmacological properties of rhIGF-I are such that it may reduce the muscle fatigue associated with PPS. Accordingly, they conducted a controlled study in 22 patients with PPS, randomized to receive either rhIGF-I at 0.05 mg/kg (n = 17) or matching placebo (n = 5) subcutaneously, twice a day for 3 months. Randomization to rhIGF-I or placebo was 3:1. The primary efficacy variables were the decline in maximal voluntary contraction (MVC) during a standardized exercise protocol and the degree of subsequent recovery within 15 min. In addition, muscle strength, metabolism as measured by magnetic resonance spectroscopy, muscle biopsy, SIP, and various rating scales for muscle fatigue were studied.

At the end of 3 months of treatment there was no difference between the two groups of patients in the degree of muscular fatigability during exercise. However, the degree of recovery of MVC within 15 min after fatiguing exercise was significantly greater ($P = 0.007$) in patients treated with rhIGF-I compared to those receiving placebo. There were no significant differences between the two groups in terms of muscle strength, morphometric analysis of muscle biopsies, fatigue, functional assessment scales, or SIP. Side effects attributable to rhIGF-I were transient and the drug was generally well tolerated. The data from this preliminary study need to be confirmed and the effects of IGF-I better defined at the molecular level. PPS represents an excellent model of a lower motor neuron syndrome that may be corrected by IGF-I treatment, sparing upper motor neuron involvement.

Myotonic Dystrophy

Myotonic dystrophy (MyD) is a multisystem autosomal dominant disorder with progressive muscle wasting and weakness demonstrated to be associated with triplet expansion [17]. In this condition, the skeletal muscle wasting and weakness is believed to be a consequence of reduced muscle protein synthesis. Associated with the skeletal muscle disorder in MyD is insulin resistance: during glucose tolerance tests, patients with MyD demonstrate marked hyperinsulinaemia. There is increasing evidence that this insulin resistance may be a causal factor in the reduced muscle protein synthesis. Attempts to bypass the insulin resistance in MyD by the administration of large doses of insulin have not been successful. IGF-I, however, may exert its insulin-like properties in insulin-resistant states. The reduction of insulin resistance by IGF-I in normal subjects and in patients with type I and type II diabetes, and the presence of IGF-I receptors in high concentrations in muscle [18] suggest a role for IGF-I in the treatment of MyD.

This possibility was explored by Vlachopapadopolou et al. [19] who assessed whether rhIGF-I could overcome the resistance to the effects of insulin on glucose and aminoacid metabolism and, at the same time, improve muscle function in patients with MyD. Patients with an established diagnosis of MyD were randomized to receive either 5 mg rhIGF-I or placebo injection subcutaneously, twice a day for 4 months. During this period the patients were maintained on a meat-free, high-protein diet. Initially, 9 patients were randomized to receive rhIGF-I and 9 to receive placebo. However, 2 patients in the rhIGF-I treated group were withdrawn from the study because of side effects. Consequently, 7 patients received rhIGF-I and 9 received placebo. Body composition, glucose and insulin metabolism, nitrogen excretion, insulin resistance, hormone levels, manual muscle strength (MMS) and functional ability were measured before and at the end of the study. In the MMS test, 34 muscle groups were tested and the results averaged. Two tests were carried out before the start of therapy to evaluate the reliability of the evaluation. The patients' perception of change in functional ability was measured by a neuromuscular function (NMF) scale designed primarily to test the motor function of peripheral muscles. Twenty-eight functional activities ranging from opening bottles to running were monitored.

Following treatment with rhIGF-I for 4 months there were statistically significant changes in body composition. Weight and lean body mass increased, body fat decreased. These changes were significantly different from those measured in the placebo treated group. Concomitantly, glucose disposal and the insulin sensitivity index increased, and urinary nitrogen decreased. Importantly, changes in skeletal muscle performance accompanied these biochemical changes. In the 7 MyD patients receiving rhIGF-I there was an increase in muscle strength at the end of the 4 months of treatment. This improvement did not reach statistical significance. However, when the data from a subset of four patients receiving greater than 70 μg/kg day were analyzed separately, a larger and statistically significant change in muscle strength was observed (Table 3).

Similarly, neuromuscular function improved in all patients receiving rhIGF-I, significantly so in those receiving greater than 70 μg/kg day (Table 4). The four patients receiving this dose showed other, more dramatic signs of improvement in muscle strength, being able to perform tasks that they had not been able to do for many years. Two severely affected patients were unable to climb stairs without holding on to the rail or to rise from a recumbent posture without support. After 4 months of rhIGF-I treatment they were able to carry out both of these tasks without any support. In addition, the systemic features of MyD improved: they had more energy, were less tired, and had improved speech and vision. Interestingly, within a month of discontinuing rhIGF-I therapy, the clinical state and neuromuscular function reverted to pre-treatment levels.

Table 3. Manual muscle strength before and at the end of 4 months treatment (with permission from [18])

	n	Manual muscle stength (mean ± sd)		
		Pre-therapy	End of therapy	Change
Placebo	9	6.90 ± 0.60	6.85 ± 0.50	0.05 ± 0.04
rhIGF-I	7	6.81 ± 0.76	7.01 ± 0.87	0.20 ± 0.31*
rhIGF-I >70 μg/kg	4	6.85 ± 0.82	7.51 ± 1.25	0.66 ± 0.29**

* $P = 0.19$; ** $P < 0.02$ change from baseline compared to placebo

Table 4. Neuromuscular function before and at the end of 4 months treatment (with permission from [18])

	n	Neuromuscular function (mean ± sd)		
		Pre-therapy	End of therapy	Change
Placebo	9	82.8 ± 17.9	85.6 ± 16.5	2.8 ± 3.4
rhIGF-I	7	80.5 ± 23.2	92.4 ± 22.5	11.9 ± 3.2*
rhIGF-I>70 μg/kg	4	74.0 ± 24.8	91.5 ± 24.0	17.5 ± 14.5**

* $P = 0.07$; ** $P < 0.02$ change from baseline compared to placebo

Thus, the study of Vlachopapadopolou et al. [19] demonstrated the beneficial effects of long-term administration of rhIGF-I on insulin sensitivity, glucose utilization, whole body protein kinetics, body composition, and muscle function in patients with MyD. Clearly, it was not possible to determine from this study the mechanism by which rhIGF-I reduced insulin resistance. However, since rhIGF-I lowered the insulin concentration without markedly lowering that of glucose, it was postulated that the improved insulin sensitivity and insulin action may be direct effects of rhIGF-I on the IGF receptor which is translated into improved insulin action. It is significant that in isolated muscle, IGF-I caused an increase in glucose and aminoacid uptake by acting on receptors for IGF-I, rather than for insulin. The increases in body weight and lean body mass with the decreases in body fat and urinary nitrogen are consistent with the increased muscle synthesis in patients receiving rhIGF-I. The translation of these biochemical changes into improved muscle strength and function is remarkable. Clearly, a further, larger study is necessary to confirm these findings and to determine the most appropriate dose. This most interesting study indicated that at least 70 μg/kg twice a day is necessary to produce significant improvements in neuromuscular function.

Duchenne Dystrophy

Duchenne muscular dystrophy (DMD) is a progressive condition inherited as an X-linked recessive trait. The condition is characterized by progressive muscular weakness, and most patients die in early adulthood. Recent studies have shown that prednisone rapidly improves the strength and function of patients with DMD although the mechanism by which the steroid exerts these effects is not known [20]. Rifai et al. [21] studied the effect of prednisone on muscle and whole body protein metabolism in six patients with DMD. The patients received prednisone at 0.75 mg/kg day (maximum dose, 40 mg/day) together with calcium carbonate. Both drugs were taken orally for 6-8 weeks. At baseline and at the end of the study period, muscle protein breakdown, fractional muscle protein synthesis and whole body protein kinetics were measured. In addition, muscle function and plasma insulin, glucagon, growth hormone and IGF-I were measured. Muscle function tests consisted of a manual muscle test (MMT) involving 26 muscle groups and maximal voluntary isometric strength using a Quantitative Muscle Testing (QMT) system. Following administration of prednisone and calcium for 6-8 weeks, there was a marked increase in muscle function. Strength improved in all patients. The average increase in strength was 13% ($P < 0.001$) as assessed by MMT and 15% ($P < 0.04$) as assessed by QMT. Associated with these changes in muscle function was an increase in muscle mass. Fractional muscle protein synthesis and whole body protein synthesis did not change significantly. Fasting plasma IGF-I concentrations increased in all patients and the mean IGF-I levels increased 80% ($P < 0.001$) from 15.4 ± 3.4 nmol/l at baseline to 27.7 ± 4.3 nmol/l after treatment. The authors concluded

that the effects of prednisone are mediated through inhibition of muscle prote-
olysis rather than stimulation of muscle protein synthesis. While the increase in
IGF-I levels was significant, the relevance of this finding to the beneficial
actions of prednisone is uncertain. Clearly, an evaluation of the efficacy of
rhIGF-I in Duchenne muscular dystrophy is now indicated.

Conclusions

Given the efficacy demonstrated for IGF-I in the few clinical conditions described
herein and the substantial body of pre-clinical evidence for a role in the central
and peripheral nervous systems, continuing research into the potential therapeutic utility of IGF-I in neurological disease is clearly justified. From a scientific
standpoint, it is important to underline that IGF-I already has a place in history,
being the first neurotrophic agent shown to be effective in ALS without being
associated with clinically relevant side effects. IGF-I is a pleiotropic molecule
active on different targets, but its mechanism of action needs to be better defined
and its ability to cross the blood-brain barrier needs to be evaluted. It is likely
that forthcoming clinical trials will evaluate the actions of this agent in other
conditions affecting the peripheral nervous system such as diabetes- and
chemotherapy-induced neuropathies.

More pre-clinical data are needed to evaluate the possibility of administer-
ing IGF-I in association with molecules demonstrated to the active on the neuromuscular system through different mechanisms of action (e.g. riluzole). The
introduction of IGF-I into the clinic may represent the first step in designing
more enlightened therapeutic strategies that will have positive effects on neuromuscular and neurodegenerative diseases in the near future.

Acknowledgements

This work was supported in part by a grant of the I.R.C.C.S. Maggiore Hospital,
Milano. We thank C.J. Jones for critically reading the manuscript.

References

1. D'Ercole AJ, Ye P, Calikoglu AS, Gutierrez-Ospina G (1996) The role of the insulin-like
    growth factors in the central nervous system. Mol Neurobiol 13:227-255
2. Radunovic A, Leigh PN on behalf of the European Familial ALS group (1996) Cu/Zn
    superoxide dismutase gene mutations in amyotrophic lateral sclerosis: correlation
    between genotype and clinical features. J Neurol Neurosurg Psychiatry 61:565-572
3. Appel SH (1981) A unifying hypothesis for the cause of amyotrophic lateral sclerosis,
    parkinsonism, and Alzheimer disease. Ann Neurol 10:499-505
4. Kerkhoff H, Hassan SM, Troost D, Van Etten RW, Veldman H, Jennekens FGI (1994)

Insulin-like and fibroblast growth factors in spinal cords, nerve roots and skeletal muscle of human controls and patients with amyotrophic lateral sclerosis. Acta Neuropathol 87:411-421

5. Braunstein GD, Reviczky AL (1987) Serum insulin-like growth factor-I levels in amyotrophic lateral sclerosis. J Neurol Neurosurg Psychiatry 50:792-794
6. Doré S, Kreiger C, Kar S, Quirion R (1996) Distribution and levels of insulin-like growth factor (IGF-I and IGF-II) and insulin receptor binding sites in the spinal cords of amyotrophic lateral sclerosis (ALS) patients. Mol Brain Res 41:128-133
7. Adem A, Ekblom J, Gillberg P-G (1994) Growth factor receptors in amyotrophic lateral sclerosis. Mol Neurobiol 9:225-231
8. Bensimon G, Lacomblez L, Meininger V, and the ALS/Riluzole Study Group (1994) A controlled trial of riluzole in amyotrophic lateral sclerosis. N Engl J Med 330:585-590
9. Lacomblez L, Bensimon G, Leigh PN, Guillet P, Meininger V for the Amyotrophic Lateral Sclerosis/Riluzole Study Group II (1996) Dose-ranging study of riluzole in amyotrophic lateral sclerosis. Lancet 347:1425-1431
10. Appel V, Stewart SS, Smith GR, Appel SH (1987) A rating scale for amyotrophic lateral sclerosis: description and preliminary experience. Ann Neurol 22:328-333
11. Lange DJ, Felice KJ, Festoff BW, Gawel MJ, Gelinas DF, Kratz R, Lai EC, Murphy MF, Natter HM, Norris FH, Rudnicki S, and the North American ALS/IGF-I Study Group (1996) Recombinant human insulin-like growth factor-I in ALS: description of a double-blind, placebo-controlled study. Neurology 47[Suppl 2]:S93-S95
12. Lai EC, Felice KJ, Festoff BW, Gawel MJ, Gelinas DF, Kratz R, Murphy MF, Natter HM, Norris FH, Rudnicki SA, and the North America ALS/IGF-I Study Group (1997) Effect of recombinant human insulin-like growth factor I (rhIGF-I) on progression of amyotrophic lateral sclerosis: a placebo-controlled study. Neurology (in press)
13. Borasio GD, De Jong JMBV, Emile J, Guiloff R, Jerusalem F, Leigh N, Murphy M, Robberecht W, Silani V, Wokke J, and the European ALS/IGF-I study group (1996) Insulin-like growth factor-I in the treatment of amyotrophic lateral sclerosis: Results of the European multicenter, double-blind, placebo-controlled trial. J Neurol [Suppl 2]:S26
14. Leigh N, and The North American and European ALS/IGF-I study groups (1997) The treatment of ALS with recombinant human insulin-like growth factor I (rhIGF-I): pooled analysis of two clinical trials. Neurology 48:A217
15. Sharma KR, Kent-Braun J, Mynhier MA, Weiner MW, Miller G (1994) Excessive muscular fatigue in the postpoliomyelitis syndrome. Neurology 44:642-646
16. Miller RG, Gelinas DF, Kent-Braun J, Dobbins T, Dao H, Dalakas M (1997) The effect of recombinant insulin like growth factor 1 (rhIGF-1) upon exercise-induced fatigue and recovery in patients with post-polio syndrome. Neurology 48:A217
17. Pizzuti A, Friedman DL, Caskey CT (1993) The myotonic dystrophy gene. Arch Neurol 50:1173-1179
18. Yu KT, Czech MP (1984) The type I insulin-like growth factor receptor mediates the rapid effects of multiplication-stimulating activity on membrane transport system in rat soleus muscle. J Biol Chem 259:3090-3095
19. Vlachopapadopoulou E, Zachwieja JJ, Gertner JM, Manzione D, Bier DM, Matthews DE, Slonim AE (1995) Metabolic and clinical response to recombinant human insulin-like growth factor I in myotonic dystrophy: A clinical research center study. J Clin Endocrinol Metab 80:3715-3723
20. Griggs RC, Moxley III RT, Mendell JR, Fenichel GM, Brooke MH, Pestronk A, Miller JP, Cwik VA, Pandya S, Robison J, King W, Signore L, Schierbecker J, Florence J, Matheson-Burden N, Wilson B (1993) Duchenne dystrophy: randomized, controlled trial of prednisone (18 months) and azathioprine (12 months). Neurology 43:520-527

21.   Rifai Z, Welle S, Moxley III RT, Lorenson M, Griggs RC (1995) Effect of prednisone on protein metabolism in Duchenne dystrophy. Am J Physiol 268 (Endocrinol Metab 31):E67-E74

Insulin-like Growth Factor-I Effects on ADP-Ribosylation Processes and Interactions with Glucocorticoids During Maturation and Differentiation of Astroglial Cells in Primary Culture

R. Avola[1], V. Spina Purrello[1], M. C. Morale[2], F. Gallo[3], Z. Farinella[3], A. Costa[1], S. Reale[1], N. Marletta[1], N. Ragusa[1], B. Marchetti[2,3]

Introduction

Nervous system function depends upon the extensive and intimate coupling between neuronal cells and glial cells [1, 2]. We have recently shown [3, 4] that during differentiation in vitro, astroglial cells in primary culture release polypeptide growth factors that exert dramatic effects on the differentiation of an immortalized hypothalamic LH-RH neuronal (Gt$_{1-1}$ subclone) cell line [3-6]. The growth factors (GFs) have emerged as crucial intercellular signaling agents that coordinate the developmental and adult physiological processes of both astrocytes and neurons [6-8]. Insulin-like growth factors I and II (IGF-I and IGF-II) are peptide growth factors structurally related to insulin. IGF-I, IGF-II and fibroblast growth factors (FGFs) are synthesized by developing astroglial cells and exert autocrine and paracrine mitogenic actions [6-9]. Primary astroglial cells possess IGF receptors and synthesize IGFs and IGF binding proteins [9, 10]. Epidermal growth factor (EGF), basic fibroblast growth factor (bFGF), IGF-I and insulin are potent mitogens capable of inducing cell division in various cell types and in particular in cultured cells from the central nervous system (CNS) [6-8, 11-13]. The effects of bFGF on the morphology of cultured astrocytes prepared from various areas of newborn rat brain, and on their expression of glial fibrillary acidic protein (GFAP) and glutamine synthetase (GS) have also been described [14]. Furthermore, EGF acts as a neurotrophic agent preferential for dopaminergic neurons in rat embryonic mesencephalic cultures [12], and enhances the proliferation of cultured astrocytes from rat brain [7, 15].

The effects of various GFs, including EGF, IGF-I, and bFGF, on macromolecular synthesis (measured by the metabolic labeling of DNA, ribosomal RNA, polyadenylated mRNA, cytoskeletal proteins, histone and non-histone proteins) in primary astroglial cell cultures have been investigated [7, 8, 15-17]. It was shown that GFs variously enhance immature astrocyte proliferation and regulate the expression of GFAP mRNA [15, 16]. Moreover, these growth factors may regulate gene expression in cultured astrocytes by an ADP-ribosylation process.

Departments of [1]Biochemistry and [3]Pharmacology, Faculty of Medicine, University of Catania, and [2]Biotech. Neuropharmacol. OASI Institute for Research and Care (IRCCS) on Mental Retardation and Brain Aging, Troina (EN), Italy

Nuclear poly-ADP ribose polymerase (pADPRP) and cytoplasmic ADP-ribosyl-transferase are the key enzymes involved in poly-ADP-ribosylation and mono-ADP-ribosylation, respectively. Recently, a marked and significant increase of pADPRP activity in bFGF or IGF-I treated fetal rat brain tissue slices was reported [17]. In addition, EGF or/and insulin treatment resulted in a dose and time dependent increase in pADPRP activity in 18-day-old rat embryo brain slices [17].

The present investigation studied the effect of growth factors (EGF, bFGF, IGF-I and insulin) on nuclear DNA and RNA synthesis in 16 days in vitro (DIV) astrocyte cultures, and on nuclear pADPRP and mitochondrial ADP-ribosyl-transferase activities, from "developing" (30 DIV) or "aging" (90 and 190 DIV) primary rat astrocyte cultures. We have also investigated the biological effects of glucocorticoid hormones and their possible interaction with GFs. Indeed, adrenal corticosteroids are known to markedly influence the astroglial cell compartment [18], and are key hormones participating in neurodegenerative changes during brain aging [19]. In astroglial cells, the glucocorticoid receptors (GRs) mediate the expression of GFAP, glutamine synthetase [18, 20], and the intermediate filament protein of astrocytes [20, 21].

Materials and Methods

Astroglial Cell Cultures

Primary astroglial cell cultures were prepared from the cerebral hemispheres of newborn rats [7, 8, 15, 22]. The meninges were removed, and the cerebral hemi-spheres were passed through a sterile nylon sieve (82 μm pore size) into nutri-ent medium. The basal nutrient medium consisted of Dulbecco's modified Eagle medium (DMEM) containing 10% heat-inactivated fetal calf serum (FCS), glutamine (2 mM), penicillin (50 U/ml) and streptomycin (50 mg/ml). The cul-tures were grown in Falcon plastic petri dishes (35, 60 or 100 mm diameter) at a plating density of 0.5-1 x 10^5 cells/cm^2 and incubated at 37°C in a humidified, 5% CO_2, 95% air atmosphere. The culture medium was changed after 7 days and then twice a week. The cell morphology of our astroglial cell cultures has been previously described [5, 7, 8].

Serum Deprivation, Growth Factor and Hormone Treatments, and Incorporation of [Methyl-³H] Thymidine

Astroglial cells were grown in serum-supplemented medium (SSM). Astroglial cells, 48 h after the last medium change, were washed in DMEM without serum and were incubated in chemically defined medium consisting of DMEM supple-mented with fatty acid-free bovine serum albumin (BSA, 1 mg/ml). Cells were deprived of serum for 24 h and then incubated for 12 h with growth factors. The following concentrations were used: IGF-I (10 ng/ml), bFGF (5 ng/ml), EGF (10 ng/ml) or insulin (10 µg/ml). [Methyl-^{3}H] thymidine (2 µCi/ml) was added to the culture medium and incubation was continued for 2 h at 37°C. At the end of the incubation, nuclei were purified as previously described [15]. Nuclear DNA labeling and RNA content were evaluated according to the method of the TRI reagent (Sigma).

To study glucocorticoid-growth factor interactions, the following compounds were used, either alone or in combination: IGF-I (10 ng/ml), bFGF (5 ng/ml), dexamethasone (10^{-9} M).

Nuclear and Mitochondrial ADP-Ribosylation Processes in Growth Factor-Treated Astrocyte Cultures

Astrocyte cultures were grown in serum-supplemented medium for 14, 28, 88 or 188 days in vitro and then switched to serum-free medium containing BSA for a 24 h starvation period before 12 h treatment with EGF (10 ng/ml), bFGF (5 ng/ml), IGF-I (10 ng/ml) or insulin (10 µg/ml). Nuclei and mitochondria were purified as previously described [15]. The assays for pADPRP activity in purified nuclei and ADP-ribosyltransferase activity in purified mitochondria were performed according to Masmoudi et al. [23].

Results

Effect of Growth Factors on Nuclear and Mitochondrial ADP-Ribosylation Processes in Developing or Aging Astrocyte Cultures

Treatment for 12 h with bFGF (5 ng/ml), IGF-I (10 ng/ml), EGF (10 ng/ml) and/or insulin (10 µg/ml) significantly stimulated nuclear DNA labeling in astrocyte cultures at 16 DIV. The order of efficacy was the following: EGF> insulin+EGF>insulin>bFGF>IGF-I. No synergistic effect was observed following the concomitant addition of EGF and insulin. Treatment with the growth factors bFGF, IGF-I, and insulin, but not EGF resulted in a marked increase in nuclear RNA content. In particular, the nuclear RNA/DNA ratio sharply increased in astrocyte cultures treated for 12 h with bFGF, IGF-I, EGF or insulin.

Nuclear poly-ADPRP activity increased sharply in 16 DIV astroglial cell cultures treated with IGF-I and bFGF (about 100% and 140%, respectively). A marked and significant increase in both nuclear pADPRP and mitochondrial ADP-ribosyltransferase in 30 DIV astrocyte cultures treated for 12 h with insulin, EGF, or both was observed.

Nuclear pADPRP (Fig. 1) and mitochondrial ADP-ribosyltransferase (ADPRT) activities were significantly higher in control, untreated astrocyte cultures at 190 DIV, compared to 90 DIV, indicating that the ADP-ribosylation process is particularly active and involved in DNA damage and repair during cell differentiation, aging or apoptosis in culture. Treatment with EGF (10 ng/ml) or insulin (10 µg/ml) for 12 h stimulated nuclear pADPRP (Fig. 1) and

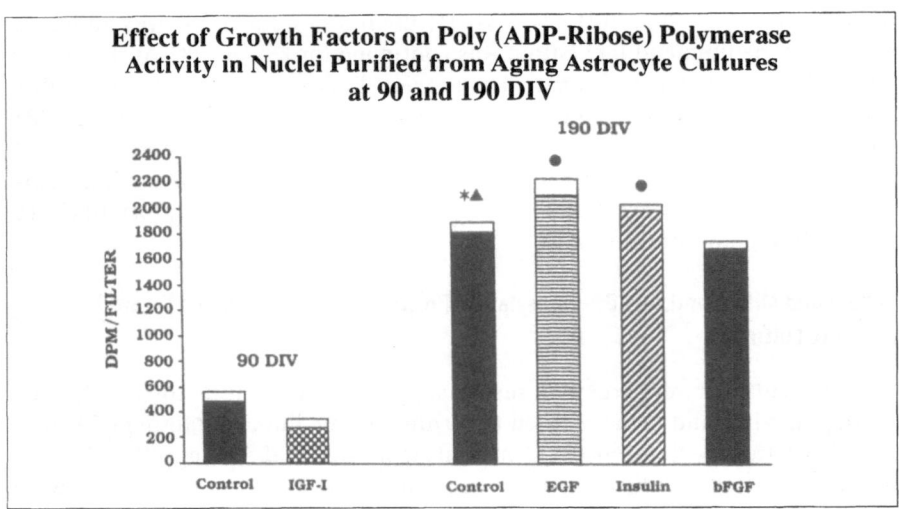

Fig.1. Effect of 12 h treatment with growth factors (bFGF, IGF-I, insulin or EGF) on poly-ADP ribose polymerase activity in nuclei purified from aging astrocyte cultures at 90 or 190 DIV. Each value is the average ± SEM of at least two independent experiments. ▫ (*white boxes*), SEM. Significance of the differences, treated vs. control, was evaluated by Student's *t*-test: ● *P*<0.05; controls at 190 DIV vs. controls at 90 DIV, ∗ ▲ *P*<0.001

mitochondrial ADPRT activities in 190 DIV aging astrocyte cultures. No significant modification of the nuclear (Fig. 1) and mitochondrial enzymes was found in 12 h IGF-I-treated astrocyte cultures at 90 DIV compared to control, untreated cultures.

Effect of Glucocorticoids, IGF-I and bFGF on DNA Labeling and Type II Glucocorticoid Receptor Expression in Developing or Aging Astrocyte Cultures

We used an in vitro model of developing neonatal rat glial cells as a first step to study the biological effects of glucocorticoids and growth factors IGF-I and bFGF, and their possible interactions. Changes in astrocyte states are likely to be responsible for changes in the extent of neurite growth, since the functional state of astroglia is critical for neurite outgrowth [2]. This work shows that the ability of astroglia to respond to glucocorticoids is a function of glia age. Expression of type II glucocorticoid receptor (GR) in developing glial cells was characterized by low levels of GR mRNA at 8 and 12 DIV, and a sharp stimulation between 20 and 50 DIV (Fig. 2a). Increases in GR mRNA levels (20-50 DIV) are accompanied by changes of astroglia morphology and proliferative activity [24]. That astroglia age is an important determinant in the effects of both glucocorticoids and GFs is supported by the finding that while young (8 DIV) astroglia respond to dexamethasone (12 h treatment) with a sharp increase in DNA labeling (Fig. 2b, c), this stimulatory effect switched to a marked inhibi-

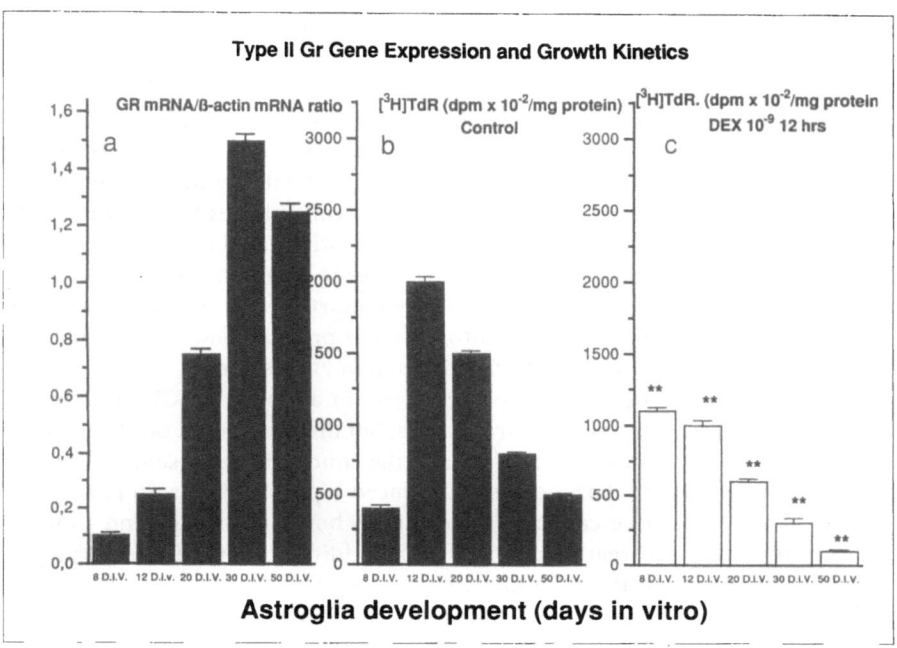

Fig.2. Glucocorticoid receptor (*GR*) gene expression and astroglial response to dexamethasone as a function of glia age. **a** Levels of GR mRNA [27] were measured during maturation of astroglial cells (8-50 DIV). **b** Astroglia proliferative capacity was evaluated by the incorporation of [^{3}H]-thymidine (*TdR*) and expressed per milligram protein. **c** Effect of dexamethasone (*DEX*) on DNA labeling as a function of a glial age. DEX induced a significant increase in proliferation at 8 DIV and a sharp inhibition at 12-50 DIV when GR levels are maximal. ∗∗ *P*< 0.01 DEX vs. control

tion in aged cultures where GR expression is maximal. In contrast, IGF-I's ability to stimulate DNA synthesis in astroglia cells appeared to increase with age [24]. Last, aged (50 DIV) glia pre-treated with IGF-I and bFGF responded to dexamethasone treatment with a marked potentiation of GF-induced proliferation [24].

Discussion

IGF-I, bFGF, EGF and insulin significantly stimulated nuclear pADPRP and mitochondrial ADP-ribosyltransferase activities in 16 and 30 DIV developing astroglial cell cultures. The sharp stimulation obtained in these primary astrocyte cultures at 30 DIV can be explained by a potentiation effect of the GFs on mitogenesis and differentiation. EGF, bFGF and insulin, but not IGF-I stimulated nuclear pADPRP and mitochondrial ADP-ribosyltransferase activities in 190 DIV, aging astrocytes. These findings may support a key role played by these growth factors in the ADP-ribosylation process involved in aging or apoptotic cell death in in vitro models.

Previously, we showed [25] that histone H1 and non-histone chromosomal proteins (NHPs) were highly ADP-ribosylated in EGF-treated fetal rat brain tissue slices. We also observed an increase of the ADP-ribosylation process in microsomal proteins after EGF treatment that correlated with the increased RNA and protein synthesis observed in astroglial cell cultures treated with EGF [15]. Cesarone et al. [26] demonstrated that EGF stimulated endogenous poly-ADPRP activity in primary rat hepatocyte cultures. The present findings indicate that EGF, insulin and bFGF may also play important and crucial roles in the post-translational modifications of chromosomal proteins and in particular in the nuclear protein ADP-ribosylation process in in vitro systems.

The morphologic and proliferative responses of astroglia to IGF-I and bFGF not only varied as a function of astroglia age, but also depended on the growth factor applied, the timing of application and the concomitant presence of glucocorticoids. In particular, dexamethasone induced biphasic effects on glial morphology and proliferative capacity, according to both culture age and time of exposure to hormonal treatment (Fig. 2). The addition of IGF-I alone sharply stimulated DNA synthesis with a magnitude depending on astroglial age, while in the presence of glucocorticoid hormones, bFGF counteracted dexamethasone-induced inhibition of DNA synthesis [25]. The fact that glucocorticoids may either act in concert with or abrogate growth factor effects at specific stages of glial differentiation supports a prominent role of glucocorticoid hormones and growth factors in maintaining cell homeostasis and astroglial cell growth regulation. Such findings indicate that glucocorticoids and growth factors interact during astroglial development and maturation in culture, suggesting a potential plasticity of the astroglial compartment to these factors during the changing environment induced by aging.

Our findings that IGF-I, EGF, bFGF and insulin stimulate nuclear DNA labeling and RNA content as well as nuclear and mitochondrial ADP-ribosylation processes in developing and aging or apoptotic astrocyte cultures indicates that these growth factors regulate and control glial development and maturation.

Acknowledgments

The help of Giuseppe Lo Re in preparing drawings and the valid collaboration and suggestions of Dr. Daniela Nici and Antonio D'Assoro in the preparation of the manuscript are gratefully acknowledged. This work was financially supported from Italian MPI and CNR.

References

1. Smith SY (1992) Do astrocytes process neural information? In: Yu ACH, Hertz L, Norenberg MD, Sykova E, Waxman SG (eds) Neuronal-astrocytic interactions.

Implications for normal and pathological CNS function. Elsevier, Amsterdam, vol 94, pp 119-136

2. Wang LC, Baird DH, Hatten ME, Mason CA (1994) Astroglial differentiation is required for support of neurite outgrowth. J Neurosci 14(5):3195-3207

3. Gallo F, Morale MC, Avola R, Marchetti B (1995) Cross-talk between luteinizing hormone-releasing hormone (LHRH) neurons and astroglial cells: developing glia release factors that accelerate neuronal differentiation and stimulate LHRH release from GT1-1 neuronal cell line and LHRH neurons induce astroglia proliferation. Endocrine 3:863-874

4. Gallo F, Morale MC, Farinella Z, Avola R, Marchetti B (1996) Growth factors released from astroglial cells in primary culture participate in the cross-talk between luteinizing hormone-releasing hormone (LHRH) neurons and astrocytes. Effects on LHRH neuronal proliferation and secretion. Ann N Y Acad Sci 784:513-516

5. Marchetti B (1996) The LHRH-astroglia network of signals as a model to study neuroimmune interactions: assessment of messenger systems, transduction mechanisms at cellular and molecular levels. Neuroimmunomodulation 3:1-27

6. Marchetti B (1997) Cross-talk signals between pathways in the CNS: Role of neurotrophic and hormonal factors, adhesion molecules and intercellular signaling agents in luteinizing hormone-releasing hormone (LHRH) neuron-astroglia interactions. Front Biosci 2:88-125

7. Avola R, Condorelli DF, Surrentino S, Turpeenoja L, Costa A, Giuffrida Stella AM (1988) Effect of epidermal growth factor and insulin on DNA, RNA and cytoskeletal protein labeling in primary rat astroglial cell cultures. J Neurosci Res 19:230-238

8. Avola R, Ragusa N, Reale S, Costa A, Insirello L, Giuffrida Stella AM (1993) Effect of growth factors (EGF, bFGF and IGF-I) on macromolecular synthesis in primary rat astroglial cell cultures. Ann N Y Acad Sci 692:192-200

9. Han VKM, Smith A, Myint W, Nygard K, Bradshaw S (1992) Mitogenic activity of epidermal growth factor on newborn astroglia: Interaction with insulin-like growth factors. Endocrinology 131:1134-1142

10. Han VKM, Lauder JM, D'Ercole EJ (1987) Characterization of somatomedin/insulin-like growth factor receptors and correlation with biological actions in cultured rat astroglial cells. J Neurosci 7:501-511

11. Morrison RS, Keating RF, Moskal JR (1988) Basic fibroblast growth factor and epidermal growth factor exert differential trophic effects on CNS neurons. J Neurosci Res 21:71-79

12. Casper D, Roboz GJ, Blum M (1994) Epidermal growth factor and basic fibroblast growth factor have independent actions on mesencephalic dopamine neurons in culture. J Neurochem 62:2166-2177

13. Rotwein P, Burgess SK, Milbrandt JD, Krause JE (1988) Differential expression of insulin-like growth factor genes in rat central nervous system. Proc Natl Acad Sci 85:265-269

14. Perraud F, Labourdette G, Eclancher F, Sensenbrenner M (1990) Primary cultures of astrocytes from different brain areas of newborn rats and effects of basic fibroblast growth factor. Dev Neurosci 12:11-21

15. Avola R, Condorelli DF, Turpeenoja L, Ingrao F, Reale S, Ragusa N, Giuffrida Stella AM (1988) Effect of epidermal growth factor on the labeling of the various RNA species and of nuclear proteins in primary rat astroglial cell cultures. J Neurosci Res 20:54-63

16. Avola R, Magrì G, Ingrao F, Insirello L, Carpano P, Nicoletti VG, Condorelli DF, Ragusa N, Giuffrida Stella AM (1991) Effect of EGF on DNA labeling in rat cerebellar imma-

ture astrocytes maintained under different culture conditions. Ann N Y Acad Sci 633:540-542

17. Avola R, Spina-Purrello V, Reale S, Costa A, Lalicata C, Ragusa N, Giuffrida Stella AM (1994) ADP-ribosylation process of nuclear protein in glial cell cultures and fetal rat brain tissue slices treated with growth factors. First European Meeting on Glial Cell Function in Health and Disease, Heidelberg, March 24-27 1994, p 52

18. Kumar S, De Vellis J (1988) Glucocorticoid-mediated functions in glial cells. In: Kunelberg HK (ed) Glial cell receptors. Raven, New York, pp 243-264

19. Mc Ewen BS, De Klark ER, Rostene W (1986) Adrenal steroid receptor and actions in the nervous system. Physiol Rev 66:1121-1128

20. Pearce B, Wilkin GP (1995) Eicosanoids, purine and hormone receptors. In: Kattenmann H, Ranosm BR (eds) Neuroglia. Oxford University Press, Oxford, pp 377-386

21. Rozovsky I, Laping NS, Teter B, O'Callaghan YP, Finch CE (1995) Transcriptional regulation of glial fibrillary acidic protein by corticosteroids in rat astrocytes in vitro is influenced by the duration of time in culture and by astrocyte-neuron interactions. Endocrinology 136:2066-2073

22. Booher J, Sensenbrenner M (1972) Growth and cultivation of dissociated neurons and glial cells from embryonic chick, rat and human brain in flask culture. Neurobiology 2:97-105

23. Masmoudi A, Islam F, Mandel P (1988) ADP-ribosylation of highly purified rat brain mitochondria. J Neurochem 51:188-193

24. Marchetti B, Gallo F, Morale MC, Cioni M, Farinella Z, Avola R (1995) Glucocorticoid-growth factor interactions during maturation and differentiation of astroglial cell in primary culture. 25th Annual Meeting Society for Neuroscience, San Diego, November 11-16 1995, vol 1, p 305

25. Spina-Purrello V, Avola R, Condorelli DF, Nicoletti VG, Insirello L, Reale S, Costa A, Ragusa N, Giuffrida Stella AM (1990) ADP-ribosylation of proteins in brain regions of rats during postnatal development. Int J Dev Neurosci 8(2):167-174

26. Cesarone CF, Scarabelli L, Giannoni P, Gallo G, Orunesu M (1990) Relationship between poly(ADP-ribose) polymerase activity and DNA synthesis in cultured hepatocytes. Biochem Biophys Res Commun 171:1043-1073

27. Morale MC, Batticane N, Gallo F, Barden N, Marchetti B (1995) Disruption of hypothalamic pituitary-adenocortical system in transgenic mice expressing type II glucocorticoid receptor antisense ribonucleic acid permanently impairs T-cell function. Endocrinology 136:3949-3960

Anti-Insulin-like Growth Factor I Antibodies Affect Locomotion and Passive Avoidance Performances in Sprague-Dawley Rats

D. Santucci[1], M. Luoni[2], A. Torsello[2], I. Branchi[1], E. E. Muller[2], E. Alleva[1]

Introduction

Insulin-like growth factor I (IGF-I) is a protein implicated in the regulation of several growth processes. Specifically, IGF-I mediates the action of growth hormone (GH) on its target organs and regulates both the release of somatostatin and GH from the hypothalamus and the release of GH and prolactin from the pituitary gland [1]. Moreover, it exerts a tissue-specific autocrine and paracrine role during the course of normal growth and differentiation [2]. IGF-I also plays a physiological role in the central nervous system (CNS) both during early development and adulthood [3-5]. Alteration in the level of IGF-I during early postnatal life is correlated with several brain dysfunctions [4]. IGF-I appears to participate in normal CNS development by regulating neuronal survival and differentiation and by stimulating glial growth [6]; postnatal synthesis of IGF-I has been detected in brain regions characterised by life-long processes of synapse formation, suggesting an additional role for this peptide in promoting and maintaining neuronal plasticity. Moreover, transgenic mice overexpressing IGF-I have significantly larger brains than controls, likely a result of increased cell size and number [7], while homozygous IGF-I (-/-) mice show reduced brain weights at 2 months of age [8].

In vivo data on exposure to growth factors (GFs) during the early postnatal phase strongly suggest that these agents influence physical and behavioural development of altricial rodents [9-11]. IGF-I affected somatic development when administered subcutaneously to developing rats [10] and early administration of IGF-I by intracerebroventricular (icv) route to mice did not grossly affect somatic or sensorimotor development while influencing ultrasonic vocalization behaviour on postnatal day (PND) 8 [12].

The present study aimed to verify whether IGF-I-Ab administration during fetal life influences rat neurobehavioural development. IGF-I-Ab was given at gestational day 16 and the somatic and sensorimotor development of pups was assessed daily until PND12. A wide range of reflexes giving a complete picture

[1]Section of Behavioural Pathophysiology, Laboratory of Pathophysiology of Organs and Systems, Istituto Superiore di Sanità, Viale Regina Elena 299, I-00161 Rome and
[2]Department of Pharmacology, University of Milan, Via Vanvitelli 32, I-20129 Milano, Italy

of the achieved level of sensorimotor maturation known as the Fox battery [13] was measured. The pattern of ultrasonic vocalization on PND3, 7, and 11 was also recorded to assess the developmental state achieved by the pups. Ultrasonic vocalizations are a useful diagnostic tool in developmental studies, as the rate of calls was found to be age-dependent in neonatal mice [14]. Moreover, learning and retention deficits were assessed at weaning by a passive-avoidance task. Levels of locomotor activity and latency time were measured on PND40 in an open field arena to investigate responses to relevant odour stimuli (social-type).

Materials and Methods

Animals

Sprague-Dawely rats were purchased from Charles River Italia (Calco, Italy). The animals were kept in an air-conditioned room at 21 ± 1°C and 60 ± 10% relative humidity, with a white/red light cycle. Males and multiparous females were housed as couples in 42x27x14 cm^3 plexiglass boxes with a metal top and sawdust bedding. Pellet food (enriched standard diet, Mucedola, Settimo Milanese, Italy) and tap water were freely available. Two weeks after arrival, 16 breeding pairs were formed and housed separately. Day 1 of pregnancy was the day in which spermatozoa were found in vaginal smears. On gestational day 16, females were treated, individually housed and inspected daily for delivery. Eight litters (4 pups each) were used in each treatment.

Anti-IGF-I Antibodies

On day 16 of gestation, pregnant rats were deeply anaesthetized with 30 mg/kg pentobarbital sodium (ip) dissolved in 1.6 ml physiological saline. After laparotomy, the uterine horns were completely withdrawn from the abdominal cavity and covered with a sterile moistened gauze. The number and the position of living fetuses were recorded. A sterile insulin needle, mounted on a Hamilton microliter syringe was carefully introduced into the amniotic cavity, passing through the placental tissues. The correct position of the needle tip was observed through the uterine wall, which is quite transparent at this stage of gestation. Each fetus received 5 µl of sheep antiserum against human IGF-I (a kind gift of Dr. B. Breier, University of Auckland, New Zealand) or 5 µl normal sheep serum. After injecting all fetuses, the uterus was repositioned into the abdominal cavity and the laparotomy was closed with silk stitches. There were no differences in reabsorption rate, number of pups born and male-to-female ratio between the experimental and control groups.

General Development and Growth (PND2 - PND15)

In each rat, reflexes and developmental hallmarks were assessed. The emergence of adult-like responses [9, 13] in a series of reflexes (righting, forelimb and hindlimb grasping, forelimb placing, vertical screen climbing) and measures of somatic growth (body weight gain, eye opening and incisor eruption) were assessed from PND2 until PND15.

Ultrasonic Vocalization (PND3, 7 and 11)

Recording of ultrasonic calls took place in a sound-attenuating chamber (Amplisilence, I-0070 Robassomero, Italy). Pups were removed from the litter and individually placed in a double-walled glass container (diameter 5 cm, height 5 cm) maintained at 25°C. Pups' axillary temperature was recorded by a temperature probe (BAT-12 Physitemp Instrument Inc, Clifton, USA). A Bruel & Kjaer (B&K, Denmark) microphone model 4135 (preamplifier B&K, 2633) was suspended 1 cm above the dish. Vocalization signals were filtered (tunable bandpass Khron-Hite filter 3500 set at 20-90 KHz), amplified (B&K Measuring Amplifier 2610), and recorded for 5 min on a Racal Store 4DS tape recorder using a direct-mode recording procedure (tape speed 76.8 cm/s). The number of ultrasonic calls emitted during the 5 min test was assessed by listening to the audible output of the tape recorder upon reduction of the tape speed to 9.6 cm/s [15, 16].

Passive Avoidance Testing (PND20 - PND21)

The avoidance apparatus (Ugo Basile, Comerio, Italy), consisted of a tilting-floor plexiglass cage divided into start and escape compartments (18x9.5x16 cm^3 each) by a sliding partition door. The start compartment was white and illuminated from above by a white light, whereas the escape compartment was black and maintained in the dark. The metallic grid floor (bars 3 mm in diameter spaced 5 mm apart) was connected to a scrambling shocker set at 0.4 mA. Avoidance tests were performed between 9:30 a.m. and 12:30 p.m., that is, during the initial portion of the light period. The procedure consisted of two phases, acquisition and retention, which took place on two consecutive days.

Acquisition Phase (PND20)

Two control and two treated pups of each litter were randomly assigned to each of the two testing conditions (conditioned and non-reinforced groups). Conditioned pups were individually placed into the start compartment facing away from the door. The sliding door between the compartments was raised, and the pup was allowed to cross into the dark chamber. When the pup crossed (4-paw criterion), lowering the tilting floor, the door shut and a 3-second 0.3 mA footshock was delivered to the grid floor. The trial ended when the rat gave the step-through response or remained in the start compartment for 120 s, which ever event occurred first. At the end of each trial, pups were removed from the apparatus and left undisturbed for a 45 s intertrial interval. The acquisition phase ended when either the subject had remained in the start compartment for two consecutive trials (learning criterion), or after 10 trials ended by stepping-through. If the learning criterion was achieved before the 10th trial, then all remaining trials (to a total of 10) were considered as 120 s latencies. Rats assigned to the non-reinforced control group were subjected to a similar multitrial session in the same apparatus, but step-through responses were not punished by foot-shock. The number of trials needed to achieve the learning criterion and the latency to step-through were used as an index of learning.

Retention Phase (PND21)

The procedure was identical for conditioned and non-reinforced pups and consisted of a single trial not punished by foot-shock. The retention trial ended when either the pup gave the step-through response or remained in the start compartment for 120 s. Latency to step-through was used as an index of retention.

Open Field Testing (PND40)

The apparatus was an open field arena (120x120x60 cm^3) made of black plexiglas, with the floor subdivided into squares 30x30 cm^2 each. At the beginning of the test, each pup was placed in one corner of the arena and his behaviour was videorecorded for 15 min. The following responses were measured by an investigator blind to the treatment: *crossing* (crossing the square limits with both forepaws); *rearing* (standing on hind legs); *wall rearing* (standing on hind legs and placing forelimbs on the wall of the arena); *grooming* (wiping, licking, combing or scratching any part of the body); and *inactivity* (no visible movements). The observational data were collected and analyzed using the software the Observer, which permitted scoring duration and frequency of each response except for crossing, for which only the frequency was measured [17]. At the end of the 20-min session, 2 petri dishes were presented to the rat in opposite corners of the arena: one dish contained sawdust bedding of a male rat; the other contained sawdust of a female. Latency time of nose contact to the dish was recorded to the neareast 0.01 s.

Statistical Analysis

A mixed-model ANOVA for repeated measures was used to analyze Fox battery, passive avoidance, ultrasonic vocalization and open field data, always considering the litter as the blocking factor and the treatment as the grouping factor [18].

Results

Data from somatic and sensorimotor development revealed no differences in the ontogenetic profile of IGF-I-Ab-treated animals when compared to controls. Treated and control rats, in fact, showed similar patterns for the time and appearance of sensorimotor reflexes and somatic parameters (Fig. 1). No differences were observed in the number of ultrasonic vocalizations on PND3, 7, and 11 (data not shown).

In the passive avoidance task, IGF-I-Ab-treated rats showed impairment in the acquisition phase. Specifically they exhibited shorter latencies to step-through (treatment x repeated measures F (1,14) = 4.21, P = 0.05) and needed a higher number of trials to reach the learning criterion (F(1,14) = 4.47, P = 0.06) (Fig. 2). No differences were observed in the retention phase.

In the open field test, IGF-I-Ab-treated adult male rats showed a reduction in locomotor activity and an increase in the frequency and duration of immobility behaviour whereas no differences were recorded in other behavioural items such as rearing and grooming (Fig. 3) or in the time to sniff the odour stimuli.

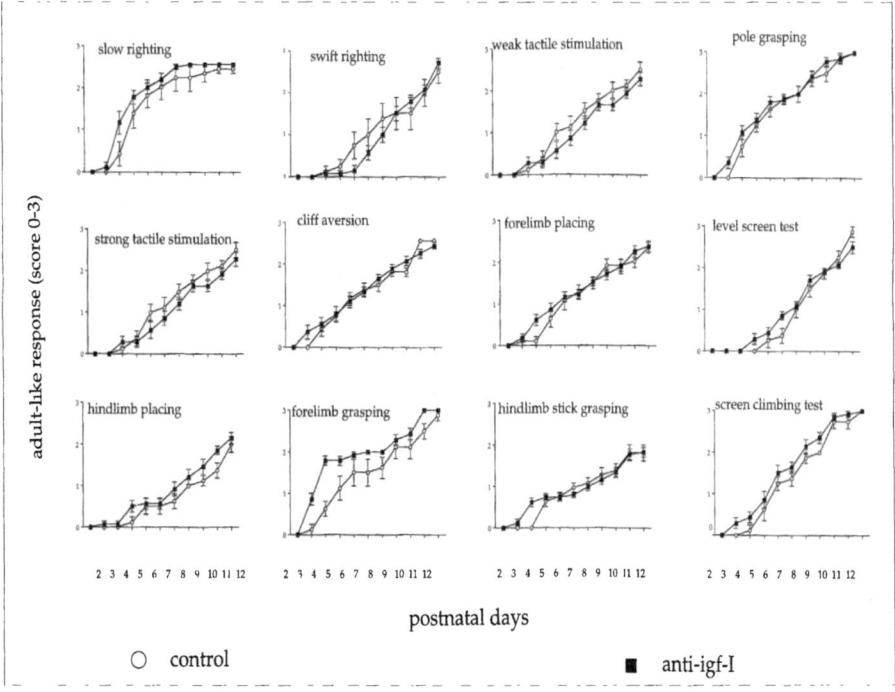

Fig. 1. Neurobehavioural data for developing anti-IGF-I-treated and control rats. Sensorimotor reflexes were assessed. Pups were scored on a scale of 0 to 3, with 3 representing an adult-like response. n = 8 in each group

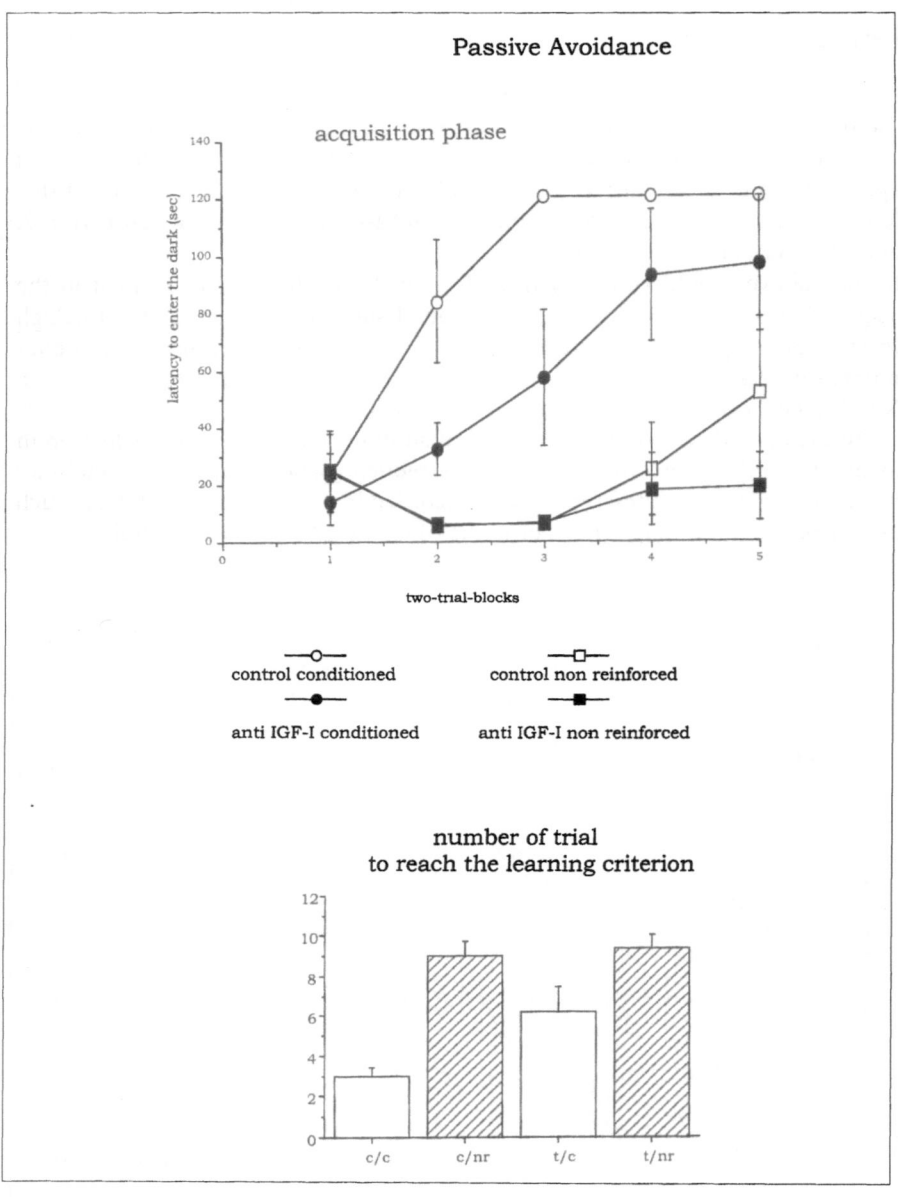

Fig. 2 a,b. Passive avoidance acquisition on PND20 in anti-IGF-I-treated and control rats. **a** Latency to enter the dark compartment in 5 blocks of two trials each. **b** Mean number of trials to reach learning criterion (±SE) in conditioned and non-reinforced pups. n = 8 in each group. c/c, control conditioned, c/nr, control non-reinforced; t/c, treated conditioned; t/nr, treated non-reinforced

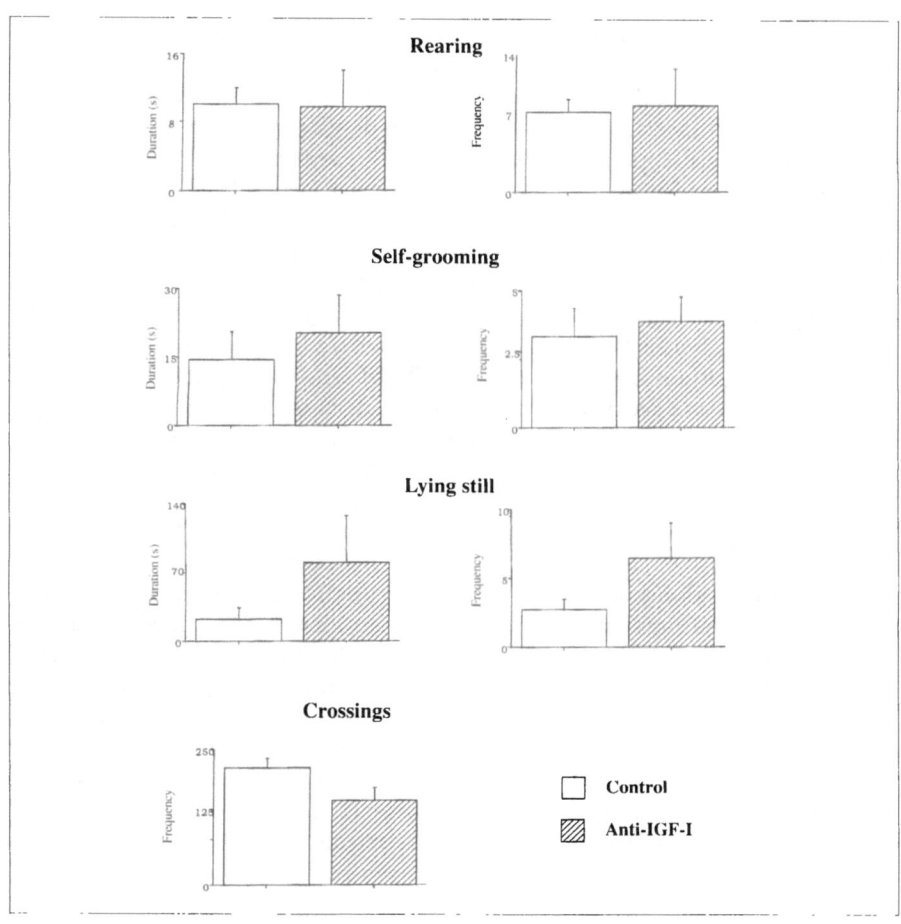

Fig. 3. Open field activity at PND40 in anti-IGF-I-treated and control rats: mean frequency and duration of rearing. Self-grooming and lyingstill; frequency of crossings. n = 8 in each group

Discussion

The present study shows that prenatal administration of a polyclonal antibody against IGF-I selectively affects the rate of acquisition of a passive avoidance task at weaning and reduces the level of locomotor activity at adulthood, while leaving unchanged somatic growth and sensorimotor development. Previous studies have shown that IGF-I administration during the early postnatal phase led to changes in both somatic and behavioural parameters measured in developing rats [10] and mice [16]. These results suggest that the time and method of administration of the growth factor, and its blockage by specific antibodies, are important variables in terms of physical and behavioural effects.

IGF-I plays a role in growth and regulation of the central nervous system and alteration of IGF-I levels during perinatal life correlates with several brain dysfunctions [4]. In the present study the antibody was administered when natural production of IGF-I peaks during fetal development. The reduced availability of this peptide might be critical by affecting brain development and neural subsystems functionality. It appears that IGF-I and IGF-II are potent trophic factors for central cholinergic neurons, and they potentially play a significant role in the differentiation, maintenance, and regeneration of these neurons [19, 20].

Interestingly, while the ontogeny of somatic and sensorimotor reflexes were not influenced by IGF-I-Ab administration, the treated rats learned the avoidance response at a significantly slower rate than did conditioned controls, as indicated by the shorter latencies to step-through and the increased number of trials needed to attain learning criterion. The absence of any difference in the behavioural performance of treated vs. control rats in the non-reinforced groups (receiving no shock) strongly suggests that the slower acquisition rate in the conditioned groups is due to associative information encoding or attentional deficit, rather than to locomotor coordination or any other side effect of the treatment (e.g. sensory impairment). Treated rats did not exhibit retention deficit. The absence of differences in retention between the treated and control reinforced pups, along with data from sensorimotor development, makes it unlikely that the groups differed in sensitivity to foot-shook. The absence of a retention deficit and the pattern of the learning slope of the acquisition phase strongly resemble those obtained from animal models of cholinergic degeneration [21] or from animals undergoing selective loss of cholinergic neurons of the basal forebrain [22]. These findings are consistent with the recent hypothesis that the cholinergic system contributes primarily to attention functions rather than to mnenic processes *per se* [23]. Moreover, in the open field arena treated adult rats were slightly less active than were controls. Reduction in activity and decreased exploratory behaviour have also been reported in rodents following neonatal cholinergic depletion [22].

Thus, an interesting working hypothesis is that alteration in endogenous levels of IGF-I at this critical time of development affects the normal course of development of neural circuitries involved in regulating cognitive function without grossly affecting somatic or behavioural development. Further investigations are necessary to evaluate the relationships between alteration in IGF-I production and developmental disorders.

Acknowledgements

This work was supported as part of the Subproject on Behavioural Pathophysiology (Project on Non-infectious Pathology) of the Istituto Superiore di Sanità and by Italian National Public Health Project "Prevention of risk factors in maternal and child health", grant 3.4.1. We are grateful to Flavia Chiarotti for expert statistical advice, Angela Valanzano and Gino de Acetis for help in treating animals and collecting experimental data, and Carla Tascone for formatting the bibliography. We thank Dr. B. Breier of the Research Center for Develop-mental Medicine and Biology, University of Auckland, for the generous gift of the anti-serum against IGF-I.

References

1. Berelowitz M, Szabo M, Frohman LA, Firestone S, Chu L, Hintz RL (1981) Somatomedin-C mediates growth hormone negative feedback by effects on both the hypothalamus and the pituitary. Science 212:1279-1281

2. Holly JMP, Wass JHA (1989) Insulin-like growth factors: autocrine paracrine or endocrine? New perspectives of the somatomedin hypothesis in the light of recent development. J Endocrinol 122:611-618

3. Baskin DG, Wilcox BJ, Figlewicz DP, Dorsa DM (1988) Insulin and insulin-like growth factors in CNS. Trends Neurosci 11:107-111

4. Sara VR, Carlsson-Skwirut C (1988) The role of insulin-like growth factors in the regulation of brain development. Prog Brain Res 73:87-99

5. Bondy CA (1991) Transient IGF-I gene expression during the maturation of functionally related central projection neurons. J Neurosci 11:3442-3455

6. Torres-Aleman I, Naftolin F, Robbins RJ (1990) Trophic effects of insulin-like growth factor-I on fetal rat hypothalamic cells in culture. Neuroscience 3:601-608

7. Carson M, Behringer RR, Brinster RL, McMorris FA (1993) Insulin-like growth factor I increases brain growth and central nervous system myelination in transgenic mice. Neuron 10:729-740

8. Beck KD, Powell-Braxton L, Widmer HR, Valverde J, Hefti F (1995) Igf1 gene disruption results in reduced brain size, CNS hypomyelination, and loss of hippocampal granule and striatal parvalbumin-containing neurons. Neuron 14:717-730

9. Alleva E, Aloe L, Calamandrei G (1987) Nerve growth factor influences neurobehavioral development of newborn mice. Neurotoxicol Teratol 9:271-275

10. Philipps AF, Persson B, Hall K, Lake M, Skottner A, Sanagen T, Sara VS (1988) The effects of biosynthetic insulin-like growth factor-I supplementation on somatic growth, maturation and erythropoiesis of the neonatal rat. Pediatr Res 23:298-305

11. Calamandrei G, Alleva E (in press) Growth factors in neurobehavioral development. In: Cosmi EV, Di Renzo GC, Hawkins DH (eds) Recent advances in perinatal medicine. Academic Publishers, London

12. Santucci D, Calamandrei G, Cagiano R (1994) IGF-I and IGF-I[24-41], but not IGF-I[57-70] affect somatic and neurobehavioral development of newborn male mice. Brain Res Bull 35:367-371

13. Fox M (1965) Reflex-ontogeny and behavioural development of the mouse. Anim Behav 13:234-241

14. Elwood RW, Keeling F (1982) Temporal organization of ultrasonic vocalization in infant mice. Dev Psychobiol 15:221-227

15. Cagiano R, Sales GD, Renna G, Racagni G, Cuomo V (1986) Ultrasonic vocalization in rat pups: effects of early postnatal exposure to haloperidol. Life Sci 38:1417-1423

16. Santucci D, Calamandrei G, Alleva E (1993) Neonatal exposure to bFGF exerts NGF-like effects on mouse behavioral development. Neurotoxicol Teratol 15:131-137

17. Noldus LP (1991) The observer: A software system for collection and analysis of observational data. Behav Res Met Inst Comp 23:415-429

18. Chiarotti F, Alleva E, Bignami G (1987) Problems of test choice and data analysis in

behavioral teratology: The case of prenatal benzodiazepines. Neurotoxicol Teratol 9:179-186

19. Knusel B, Michel PP, Schwaber JS, Hefti F (1990) Selective and nonselective stimulation of central cholinergic and dopaminergic development in vitro by nerve growth factor, basic fibroblast growth factor, epidermal growth factor, insulin and the insulin-like growth factors I and II. J Neurosci 10:558-570

20. Konishi Y, Takahashi K, Chui DH, Rosenfeld RG, Himeno M, Tabira T. (1994) Insulin-like growth factor II promotes in vitro cholinergic development of mouse septal neurons: comparison with the effect of insulin-like growth factor I. Brain Res 649:53-61

21. Holtzman DM, Santucci D, Kilbridge J, Couzens JC, Fontana DJ, Daniels SE, Johnson RM, Chen K, Sun Y, Carlson E, Alleva E, Epstein CJ, Mobley WC (1996) Developmental abnormalities and age-related neurodegeneration in a mouse model of Down syndrome. Proc Natl Acad Sci USA 93:13333-13338

22. Ricceri L, Calamandrei G, Berger-Sweeney J (1997) Different effects of postnatal day 1 vs 7 192 IgG saporin lesions on learning, exploratory behavior and neurochemistry in juvenile rats. Behav Neurosci (in press)

23. Everitt BJ, Robbins TW (1997) Central cholinergic systems and cognition. Annu Rev Psychol 48:649-684

Neuroprotective Effect of GPE Pretreatment on Rat Hippocampal Organotypic Cultures Exposed to NMDA

L. Curatolo, G. L. Raimondi, C. Caccia, E. Wong, S. Gatti, C. Post

Introduction

Insulin-like growth factor I (IGF-I), a 70 aminoacid-long polypeptide with several metabolic and proliferative actions, is expressed in the rat brain during development and after acute injury [1-3]. The neuroprotective effect of IGF-I has been recently demonstrated in vitro using differentiated PC12 cells undergoing apoptosis [4], cerebellar granules cultured in the presence of low K^+ concentrations [5], and primary rat hippocampal neurons [6]. Moreover, there is a growing body of evidence showing that IGF-I injected intracerebroventricularly (icv) is neuroprotective in several experimental models of acute neuronal injury [7-8]. This suggests a possible therapeutic use for this trophic factor in peripheral or central nerve injuries. Some of the biological effects of IGF-I are probably mediated by des(1-3)IGF-I, an IGF-I derivative lacking the N-terminal tripeptide glycine-proline-glutamate (GPE). Des(1-3)IGF-I has been detected in the human brain (among other tissues) and is generally more potent than IGF-I in several in vitro assays [9-12]. The recent observation of Guan et al. that des(1-3)IGF-I is less effective then recombinant human IGF-I (rhIGF-I) as a neuronal rescue agent suggests that the central effects of this growth factor might be partially mediated by the N-terminal tripeptide GPE [13]. GPE (10^{-5} M) exhibits in vitro mitogenic properties on glial cells [14], modifies gonadotropin releasing hormone in response to N-methyl-d-aspartate (NMDA) receptor agonists [15-16] and potentiates K^+-induced dopamine release from rat striatal slices [17]. All these effects probably involve NMDA receptor-mediated events, since they can be reverted by specific NMDA receptor antagonists.

We used an in vitro model of NMDA-induced neurodegeneration, organotypic cultures of rat hippocampus, to study the effects of GPE pretreatment on excitotoxic neuronal damage. Organotypic cultures of newborn rat hippocampus represent an interesting tool for in vitro studies since the hippocampal cytoarchitecture is maintained and the neuronal damage induced by cytotoxic agents or physical/chemical injuries is similar to that observed in vivo [18-19]. GPE's neuroprotective effect was compared to those of rhIGF-I and MK801, a well-known non-competitive NMDA antagonist.

CNS Research Biology, Pharmacia & Upjohn, Viale Pasteur 10, 20014 Nerviano (MI), Italy

Materials and Methods

GPE (supplied as 36% w/v ammonium trifluoroacetate salt) was obtained from Pharmacia & Upjohn (Stockholm, Sweden). All reagents were from Sigma (St. Louis, MO) if not otherwise indicated. The culture medium was MEM (Gibco Laboratories, Grand Island, NY) supplemented with 25% (v/v) heat-inactivated, defined horse serum (Hyclone, Logan, Utah), l-glutamine (2 mM), HEPES (15 mM), penicillin (100 U/ml), streptomycin (100 µg/ml) and glucose (5.5 mg/ml) (complete medium). Rat hippocampal organotypic cultures were prepared as described by Stoppini et al. [18, 19]. Briefly, newborn rats (6-8-days-old) were killed by decapitation under light ether anesthesia; hippocampal areas were dissected and sliced (400 µm sections). The slices were placed on a semiporous membrane (0.4 µm, Millicel-CM, Millipore, Bedford, MA) and cultured for 20 days in the presence of complete medium. Treatments were performed by replacing the culture medium with Locke's saline solution (5 mM KCl) containing either 30 µM MK801 (RBI, Natick, MA) or increasing concentrations of GPE (1-200 µM) or of rhIGF-I (Boehringer Mannheim GmbH, Germany; 1 U = 5 ng/ml).

After 30 min of preincubation, NMDA (100 µ) was added to the culture medium; after an additional 30 min of exposure, the slices were allowed to recover for 22 h in conditioned culture medium. Control cultures were incubated in Locke's saline solution containing increasing concentrations of ammonium trifluoacetate. Neuronal damage was analyzed by incubating the slices for 2 h in the presence of propidium iodide (25 µg/ml) (Calbiochem, La Jolla CA). The degree of fluorescent emission obtained when exposing the slices to a fluorescent lamp (Axiovert-10 microscope, Zeiss, West Germany) was analyzed using the Image Pro Plus software (Media Cybernetics, Silver Spring, MD). A semiquantitative measurement of neuronal damage was calculated by defining, in each experiment, the NMDA-induced cell damage as 100% relative cell damage and the control treatment (Locke's solution) as 0% relative cell damage.

Results and Discussion

In our experimental conditions the exposure of hippocampal organotypic cultures to one pulse of NMDA (30, 100, 300 µM) for 30 min caused a concentration-dependent increase in cellular damage, with a reproducible and almost maximal effect observed with 100 µM NMDA. Therefore, 100 µM NMDA was chosen as a standard neurotoxic condition for further experiments of neuroprotection. Pretreatment (30 min before NMDA) with 10 and 50 µM MK801 completely blocked NMDA-induced damage (not shown). Thus, MK801 (30 µM) was used as positive control in the experimental protocol to test GPE and rhIGF-I as neuroprotectant agents.

The neuroprotective effect of pretreatment with increasing concentrations of GPE (1-100 µM) on the NMDA-induced cellular damage is shown in Fig. 1.

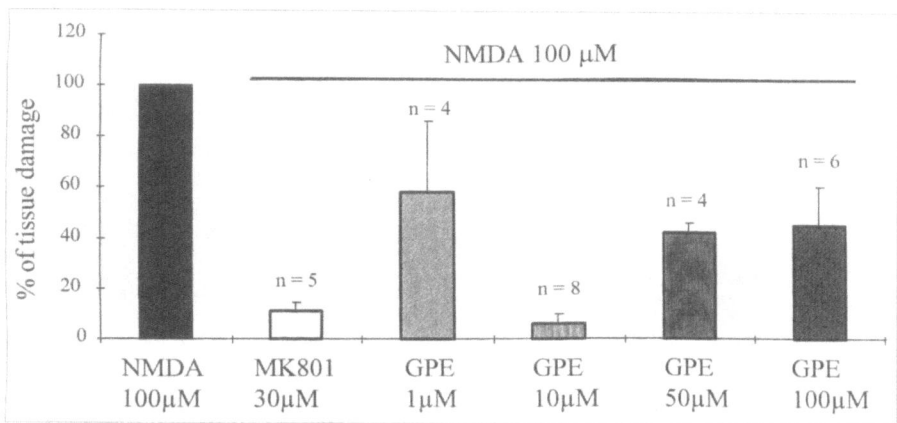

Fig. 1. Neuroprotective effect of GPE pretreatment on NMDA-induced cell damage in organotypic cultures of rat hippocampus. Results are shown as percentage of cell damage. Data are mean +/- SE obtained from 3 independent experiments

All tested concentrations significantly reduced the NMDA-induced cellular damage and the effect did not seem to be clearly concentration-dependent. The highest degree of neuroprotection (almost complete) was always obtained with 10 μM GPE while lower (1 μM) or higher (50-100 μM) concentrations always reduced the neuronal damage to a lesser extent. Direct toxicity, either of GPE (up to a concentration of 200 μM) or of ammonium trifluoroacetate (corresponding dilutions of the 36% (w/v) solution), was never observed (not shown). In addition, pretreatment with ammonium trifluoroacetate did not reduce the NMDA-induced cellular damage in our experimental conditions (not shown). Preliminary experiments using 100 nM GPE showed that the tripeptide still exerted a neuroprotectant effect at this concentration, suggesting that further studies should be performed in order to fully characterize the effect of GPE-pretreatment in our experimental model.

Pretreatment with increasing concentrations of rhIGF-I (10 nM-10 μM) in the same experimental conditions gave a significant neuroprotective effect, reaching a maximum (40% neuroprotection) at 100 nM (Fig. 2). A similar degree of neuroprotection was in fact observed with higher concentrations of rhIGF-I (1 μM and 10 μM) while the lower concentration tested (10 nM) did not reduce cellular damage significantly.

Although further studies are required to better compare the three different neuroprotectant agents and to attempt a comparative study of the different mechanisms of action, analysis of the reported data allows a few interesting remarks. GPE (10 μM) blocks completely the NMDA-induced cellular damage, as does MK801, and at similar concentrations (30 μM). However the lack of a concentration-dependent effect, at least in the considered range of concentrations, does not imply a single receptor-mediated effect. Moreover, the bell-shaped curve describing the pharmacological effect of increasing concentra-

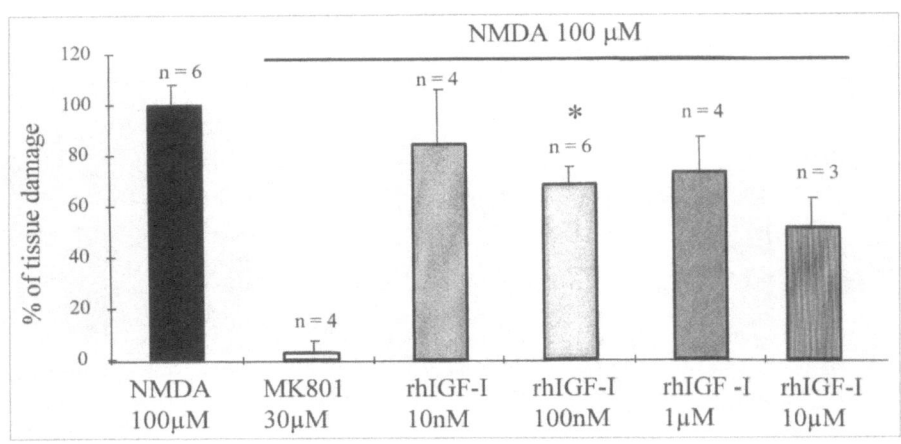

Fig. 2. Neuroprotective effect of rhIGF-I pretreatment on NMDA-induced cell damage in organotypic cultures of rat hippocampus. Results are shown as percentage of cell damage. Data are mean +/- SE obtained from one experiment representative of three. *, $P < 0.01$ vs. 100 μM NMDA in the Student's t-test

tions of GPE in our experimental model might be the result of multiple mechanisms of action. This was already suggested by Stoppini et al. [17] who demonstrated that GPE at 10^{-10} to 10^{-8} M increased the K$^+$-induced acetylcholine release from brain cortex while GPE at 10^{-10} to 10^{-4} M increased the K$^+$-induced dopamine release from rat striatum; only the latter effect was blocked by AP-7, a competitive NMDA antagonist. However, our data suggest a functional antagonism of GPE against NMDA-induced cell damage, at least in a protocol of pretreatment. Further studies investigating the possible synergism of GPE and MK801 as neuroprotectant agents in our experimental model would add another interesting piece of information about the pharmacological properties of GPE. Recombinant hIGF-I used in the same experimental conditions exhibited a lower efficiency as neuroprotective agent towards the NMDA-induced neuronal damage at any of the tested concentrations.

A final observation is related to the one-pulse exposure to NMDA and the different pharmacological agents: we have chosen this experimental protocol because the main purpose of this study was the analysis of the GPE effect on the NMDA-induced cellular damage. However this may not be a correct protocol for studies of the neuroprotective actions of IGF-I. In fact, recent in vivo data show that IGF-I is neuroprotective even when injected icv 2 h after an hypoxic/ischemic insult [7, 8]. Therefore IGF-I could be better considered to be a rescue agent. It would be interesting to test its ability to reduce the neuronal damage caused by one pulse of NMDA in organotypic cultures using a protocol of post-treatment. Further studies addressing the possibility of a direct interaction of GPE at the NMDA receptor are presently on-going in our department.

Acknowledgments

The authors are grateful to L. Benatti for useful discussion of the results and critical reading of the manuscript, and to L. Stoppini for his precious support in culture setting up.

References

1. D'Ercole AJ, Ye P, Calikoglu AS, Gutierrez-Ospina G (1996) The role of insulin-like growth factors in the central nervous system. Mol Neurobiol 13:227-255
2. Breese CR, DaCosta A, Rollins YD, Adams C, Booze RM, Sonntag WE, Leonard S (1996) Expression of insulin like growth factor I and IGF-binding protein 2 in the hippocampus following a cytotoxic lesion in the dentate gyrus. J Comp Neurol 369:388-404
3. Sandberg Norquist AC, Von Holst H, Holmin S, Sara VR, Bellander BM, Schalling M (1996) Increase of insulin-like growth factor (IGF)-1, IGF binding protein-2 and -4 mRNAs following cerebral contusion. Brain Res Mol Brain Res 38:285-293
4. Piarrizas M, Saltiel AR, Leroith D (1997) Insulin like growth factor I inhibits apoptosis using the phosphatidylinositol 3'kinase and mitogen-activated protein kinase pathways. J Biol Chem 272:154-61
5. DeMello SR, Borodezt K, Soltoff SP (1997) Insulin-like growth factor and potassium depolarisation maintain neuronal survival by distinct pathways: possible involvement of PI3 kinase in IGF-I signalling. J Neurosci 17:1548-1560
6. Lindholm D, Hughes RA, Thoenen H (1995) Multiple neurotrophic factors promote survival of central nervous system neurons. In: Ottoson D, Bartfai T, Hokfelt T, Fuxe K (eds) Challenges and perspectives in neurosciences. Wenner-Gren international series, vol 66. Pergamon, Oxford, pp 141-154
7. Guan J, Williams C, Gunning M, Mallard C, Gluckman P (1993) The effects of IGF-I treatment after hypoxic-ischemic brain injury in adult rats. J Cereb Blood Flow Metab 13:609-16
8. Johnston BM, Mallard EC Williams CE, Gluckman PD (1996) Insulin like growth factor- 1 is a potent neuronal rescue agent after hypoxic-ischemic injury in fetal lambs. J Clin Invest 97:300-8
9. Yamamoto H, Murphy LJ (1995) Enzymatic conversion of IGF-I to des(1-3)IGF-I in rat serum and tissues: a further potential site of growth hormone regulation of IGF-I action. J Endocrinol 146:141-8
10. Ballard FJ, Wallace JC, Francis GL, Read LC, Tomas FM (1996) Des(1-3)IGF-I: a truncated form of insulin-like growth factor I. Int J Biochem Cell Biol 28:1085-7
11. Zhao X, McBride BW, Trouten-Radford LM, Burton JH (1993) Effects of insulin-like growth factor I and its analogues on bovine hydrogen peroxide release by neutrophils and blastogenesis by mononuclear cells. J Endocrinol 139:259-65
12. Russo VC, Werther GA (1994) Des(1-3)IGF-I potently enhances differentiated cell growth in olfactory bulb organ culture. Growth Factors 11:301-311
13. Guan J, Williams CE, Skinner SJ, Mallard EC, Gluckman PD (1996) The effects of IGF-1, IGF-2 and des-IGF-1 on neuronal loss after hypoxic-ischemic brain injury in adult rats: evidence for a role for IGF binding proteins. Endocrinology 137:893-8
14. Ikeda T, Waldbillig RJ, Puro DG (1995) Truncation of IGF-I yields two mitogens for retinal Muller glial cells. Brain Res 686:87-92

15. Bourguignon JP, Gerard A, Alvarez Gonzalez ML, Franchimont P (1993) Acute suppression of gonadotropin-releasing hormone secretion by insulin-like growth factor I and subproducts: an age dependent endocrine effect. Neuroendocrinology 58:525-30

16. Bourguignon JP, Alvarez-Gonzalez ML, Gerard A, Franchimont P (1994) Gonadotropin releasing hormone inhibitory autofeedback by subproducts antagonist at NMDA receptors: a model of autocrine regulation of peptide secretion. Endocrinology 134:1589-92

17. Sara VR, Carlson-Skirut C, Bergman T, Jornvall H, Roberts PJ, Crawford M, Nilsson Hakansson L, Civalero I, Nordberg A (1989) Identification of Gly-Pro-Glu (GPE) the aminoterminal of insulin-like growth factor 1 which is truncated in brain, as a novel neuroactive peptide. Biochem Biophys Res Commun 165:766-771

18. Stoppini L, Buchs PA, Muller D (1991) A simple method for organotypic cultures of nervous tissue. J Neurosci Methods 37:173-182

19. Stoppini L, Buchs PA, Muller D (1993) Lesion-induced neurite sprouting and synapse formation in hippocampal organotypic cultures. Neuroscience 57:985-994

Expression of IGF-I and IGF-I Receptor mRNA in Sural Nerves of Diabetic Patients

M. Grandis[1], L. Nobbio[1], G. L. Mancardi[1], M. Abbruzzese[1], F. Maritato[2], L. Banchi[1], A. Schenone[1]

Introduction

The insulin-like growth factors (IGF-I, IGF-II) are polypeptides with both; growth-promoting and insulin-like metabolic activities [1]. IGFs, whose expression is considerable in the developing nervous system [2], have neurotrophic actions in motor [3], sensory [3] and sympathetic neurons [3-4]. Since these neural populations result to be damaged in diabetic neuropathy, it has been proposed that a loss of IGFs may be involved in the pathogenesis of this common complication of diabetes.

Previous studies, performed in rats with experimental diabetes induced by streptozotocin, demonstrated that in different tissues [5] including sciatic nerves [6], IGF-I and IGF-II mRNA abundance was significantly decreased. Moreover, there is evidence of reduced IGF-I circulating levels and impaired IGF-I receptor expression per red cell in diabetic patients with neuropathy [7]. However, to demonstrate the involvement of a trophic factor deficiency in the aetiology of a peripheral neuropathy, a reduced expression of the molecule should be observed in peripheral nerves [8]. The importance of studies conducted on diabetic patients derives also from the fact that experimental models of diabetes are almost all models of insulin-dependent diabetes mellitus (IDDM), while in human pathology non-insulin-dependent diabetes mellitus (NIDDM) is far more frequent.

By semiquantitative reverse transcriptase polymerase chain reaction (RT-PCR), we studied the expression of mRNA for IGF-I and for its receptor in sural nerves from diabetic and non-diabetic patients with peripheral neuropathy and from normal controls. Expression of IGF-I, but not of its receptor was significantly reduced in diabetic patients compared to normal controls. Our results suggest that IGF-I may be involved in the pathogenesis of human diabetic neuropathy, and introduce IGF-I as a possible therapeutic factor for this common peripheral nerve disease.

[1]Department of Neurological Sciences and Neurorehabilitation, and [2]Institute of Surgical Anatomy, University of Genoa, Via de Toni 5, 16132 Genova, Italy

Material and Methods

Patients and Sural Nerve Biopsy

Sural nerve biopsies were performed for diagnostic purposes, according to previously published techniques [9], in 6 patients affected by diabetic neuropathy (5 NIDDM, 1 IDDM), in 5 patients affected by peripheral neuropathy of the axonal type (1 vasculitic neuropathy, 2 toxic-metabolic neuropathies and 2 cases of axonal neuropathies of undetermined origin), and 4 normal controls. The normal controls were patients suspected of having peripheral neuropathy, but whose nerves upon biopsy resulted to be normal from morphologic and morphometric criteria.

Sural nerves were biopsied under local anesthesia at midcalf. Samples were fixed with 2.5% glutaraldehyde in cacodilate buffer, pH 7.4, for 2 h, and then post-fixed with 1% osmium tetroxide, in cacodilate buffer, pH 7.4, for 1 h; finally they were embedded in epon and semithin sections were prepared for morphological examination. A segment of the nerve was processed for teased fibers examination. Specimens for RNA isolation were snap-frozen in liquid nitrogen and stored at -80°C until used.

Molecular Biology

A semiquantitative RT-PCR technique was used to evaluate relative levels of IGF-I and IGF-I receptor mRNA. Briefly, total RNA was isolated from biopsied sural nerves by a single-step method (Tripure, Boheringer Mannheim, Indianapolis, IN, USA) and quantitated by spectrophotometry at 260 nm. After first strand cDNA synthesis from 500 ng total RNA, semiquantitative PCR was carried out by coamplification of IGF-I or IGF-I receptor with glyceraldehyde 3-phosphate dehydrogenase (GAPDH) as an endogenous standard sequence (Table 1). PCR was performed in 25 µl final volume containing 10 µl of the RT reaction, 1x PCR buffer (containing $MgCl_2$), 0.125 mM dNTPs (Pharmacia LKB, Piscataway, NJ, USA), 0.15 µM of each sense and antisense primer (Tib Molbiol, Genova, Italy) and 5 U native Taq polymerase (Perkin Elmer, Foster City, CA, USA). Amplification following hot start (5 min at 95°C) was carried out for 30 cycles consisting of 1 min at 95°C, 2 min at 60°C (IGF-I) or 2 min at 53°C (IGF-I receptor), and 3 min at 72°C (both). An additional extension time of 10 min at 72°C was added at the end. PCR products were analyzed on 2.0% agarose gels; band intensity, measured directly by Gel Doc 1000 System (Bio-Rad Laboratories, Milano), was used to evaluate the amount of each mRNA expressed as absolute level and as ratio between target sequence (IGF-I or IGF-I receptor) and GAPDH (relative level).

Statistical Analysis

Data were expressed as mean ± standard deviation. Analysis of variance (ANOVA) was used to compare results from the three groups, and a post-test

Table 1. Oligonucleotide primer sets used in PCR amplification

	Localization 3' end	Primer sequence	Amplified product (bp)
IGF-I	361	GGTGGATGCTCTTCAGTTCGTG	435
	749	GTGTATTTCATTGGGGGAAACGCC	
IGF-I receptor	2448	GCCTTTCACATTGTACCGCATC	600
	3001	CTCCCACTCATCAGGAACGTACAC	
GAPDH	849	TGATGACATCAAGAAGGTGGTGAAG	240
	1064	TCCTTGGAGGCCATGTGGGCCAT	

(Bonferroni t-test) was used, when appropriate, to compare the differences between the diabetic group and either normal controls or the diseased non-diabetic group.

Results

The semiquantitative RT-PCR, performed by amplifing together IGF-I and GAPDH, confirmed that IGF-I is expressed in human sural nerves. A significant reduction ($P<0.05$) of absolute levels of IGF-I mRNA in diabetic patients (612.83 ± 259.14) compared with either normal controls (1115.5 ± 261.39) or patients with axonal neuropathy (1105.4 ± 456.02), was observed. Relative levels of mRNA for IGF-I (Fig. 1A) were also decreased in diabetic patients as compared to normal controls (3.3 ± 0.9 vs. 4.9 ± 0.9; $P<0.05$) and axonal neuropathies (3.3 ± 0.9 vs. 5.0 ± 1.5; P: not significant).

The amplification of IGF-I receptor mRNA was also successful. A significant ($P<0.05$) reduction of absolute levels of mRNA for IGF-I receptor in patients with diabetic neuropathy (441.20 ± 301.00), as compared to both normal controls (881.75 ± 262.56) and axonal neuropathies (931.60 ± 209.27) was observed. However relative levels of IGF-I receptor mRNA in patients with diabetic neuropathy (Fig. 1B) were not significantly reduced when compared to normal controls (2.9 ± 0.7 vs. 3.7 ± 0.46; P: n.s.), while they appeared to be even slightly augmented when compared to the axonal neuropathies (2.9 ± 0.7 vs. 2.8 0.4; P: not significant).

Discussion

Peripheral neuropathy is a common, frequently disabling complication of diabetes [10]. In the Rochester Diabetic Neuropathy Study 59% of NIDDM patients

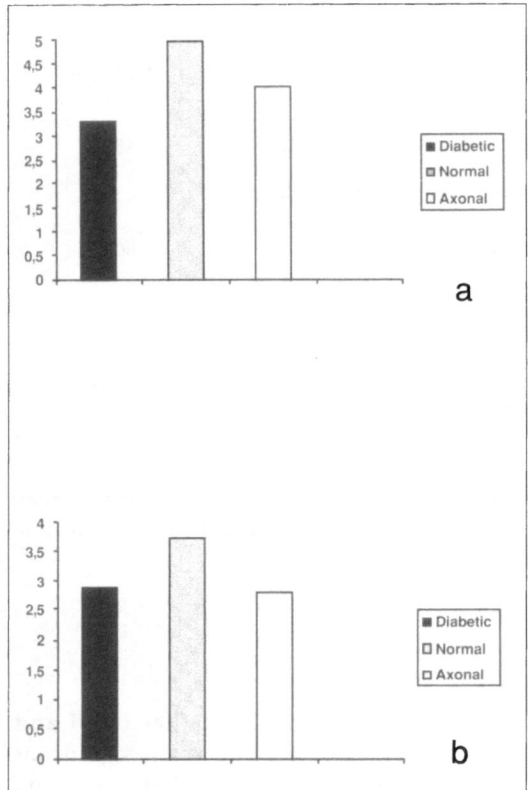

Fig. 1. Relative levels of IGF-I mRNA (**a**) were significantly lower (*P*<0.05) in diabetic patients compared to normal controls. Relative levels of IGF-I receptor mRNA (**b**) did not differ between diabetic patients and either normal or diseased controls (*axonal*)

and 66% of IDDM patients had neuropathy [11-12]. While the presence of neuropathy is certainly related to the diabetic state and to the degree of hyperglycemia, other specific metabolic and vascular abnormalities may be involved in the pathogenesis of diabetic neuropathy [13-14]. It is also unclear whether the primary effects of these metabolic and/or vascular abnormalities are on sensory neurons, on Schwann cells, or on both [15-16].

In the last years a growing body of research, mainly from STZ-treated rats [17], suggests the probable involvement of growth factors (neurotrophins, insulin-like and cytokine-like growth factors) in the pathogenesis of this frequent peripheral nervous system disease. We demonstrated by RT-PCR that IGF-I mRNA is reduced in sural nerves of patients with diabetic neuropathy, compared to both normal and diseased controls. Relative levels of IGF-I receptor mRNA in sural nerves of diabetic patients with neuropathy were not significantly impaired. In peripheral nerves of experimental diabetic rats, a significant underexpression of IGF-I mRNA was previously demonstrated [6]; moreover levels of IGF-I and IGF-I receptor mRNA per red cell were decreased in diabetic patients with neuropathy [7]. Based on these findings, IGF-I has been proposed to be involved in the pathogenesis of diabetic neuropathy [17]. Our data, showing IGF-I underexpression in the target tissue of this frequent complication of diabetes, suggest the direct involvement of IGF-I in the pathogenesis of diabetic neuropathy. Moreover, since IGF-I stimulates peripheral nerve repair [18] and is upregulated in rat sciatic nerves after transection [19], the underexpression of IGF-I in human diabetic nerves may be responsible for the defective regeneration of peripheral nerves in diabetes [16].

The observation that expression of the IGF-I receptor is relatively conserved in sural nerves of patients with diabetic neuropathy, along with the underexpression of IGF-I, suggests a possible therapeutical use of IGF-I in this complication of diabetes in order to improve the clinical features or prevent the progression of this neuropathy.

References

1. Martin DM, Yee D, Feldman EL (1992) Gene expression of the insulin-like growth factors and their receptors in cultured human retinal pigment epithelial cells. Brain Res Mol Brain Res 12(1-3):181-6
2. Beck F, Samani NJ, Byrne S et al (1988) Histochemical localization of IGF-I and IGF-II mRNA in the rat between birth and adulthood. Development 104:29-39
3. Ishii DN, Glazner GW, Pu SF (1994) Role of insulin-like growth factors in the peripheral nerve regeneration. Pharmacol Ther 62:125-144
4. Zackenfels K, Oppenheim RW, Rohrer H (1995) Evidence for an important role of IGF-I and IGF-II for the early development of chick sympathetic neurons. Neuron 14:731-741
5. Ishii DN, Guertin DM, Whalen LR (1994) Reduced insulin-like growth factor-I mRNA content in liver, adrenal glands and spinal cord of diabetic rats. Diabetologia 37:1073-1081
6. Wuarin L, Guertin DM, Ishii DN (1994) Early reduction in insulin-like growth factor gene expression in diabetic nerve. Exp Neurol 130:106-114
7. Migdalis IN, Kalogeropoulou K, Kalantzis L, et al (1995) Insulin-like growth factor-I and IGF-I receptors in diabetic patients with neuropathy. Diabet Med 12:823-827
8. Tomlinson DR, Fernyhough P, Diemel LT (1996) Neurotrophins and peripheral neuropathy. Philos Trans R Soc Lond 351:455-462
9. Dyck PJ, Giannini C, Lais A (1993) Pathological alterations of nerves. In: Dyck PJ, Thomas PK, Griffin JW, Low PA, Poduslo JF (eds) Peripheral neuropathy, 3rd ed. WB Saunders, Philadelphia, pp 514-595
10. Thomas PK, Tomlinson DR (1993) Diabetic and hypoglycemic neuropathy. In: Dyck PJ, Thomas PK, Griffin JW, Low PA, Poduslo JF, (eds) Peripheral neuropathy, 3rd edn. WB Saunders, Philadelphia, pp 1219-1250
11. Dyck PJ, Karnes JL, O'Brien PC (1992) The Rochester Diabetic Neuropathy Study: reassessment of tests and criteria for diagnosis and staged severity. Neurology 42:1164-117.
12. Dyck PJ, Litchy WJ, Lehman KA et al (1995) Variables influencing neuropathic endpoints: The Rochester Diabetic Neuropathy Study of Healthy Subjects. Neurology 45:1115-1121
13. Greene DA, Sima AAF, Pfeifer MA et al (1990) Diabetic neuropathy. Ann Rev Med 41:303-317
14. Llewelyn JG (1995) Diabetic neuropathy. Curr Opin Neurol 8:364-366
15. Scarpini E, Doronzo R, Baron P et al (1992) Phenotypic and proliferative properties

of Schwann cells from nerves of diabetic patients. Int J Clin Pharmacol Res XII (5/6):211-215

16. Bradley Jl, Thomas PK, King RHM et al (1995) Myelinated nerve fibre regeneration in diabetic sensory polyneuropathy: correlation with type of diabetes. Acta Neuropathol 90:403-410

17. Ishii DN (1995) Implication of insulin-like growth-factors in the pathogenesis of diabetic neuropathy. Brain Res Rev 20:47-67

18. Kanje M, Skottner A, Sjoberg J et al (1989) Insulin-like growth factor I (IGF-I) stimulates regeneration of the rat sciatic nerve. Brain Res 486(2):396-8

19. Cheng HL, Randolph A, Feldman EL et al (1996) Characterization of insulin-like growth factor-I and its receptor and binding proteins in transected nerves and cultured Schwann cells. J Neurochem 66:525-537

Subjects Index

Acquisition phase, 137
Adenosine
   anti-apoptotic action in CGCs, 61
Aging
   hippocampus and cognitive decline, 50
ALS (see Amyotrophic lateral sclerosis)
Alzheimer's disease, 55, 56
Amniotic cavity
   IGF-I antibodies, 136
Amyotrophic lateral sclerosis (ALS)
   effects of GAGs, 86
   effects of IGF-I, 86
   generalities, 115
   multicentre studies, 116-119
   pre-clinical studies, 85, 110, 116
Antioxidants, 64
Apoptosis
   death effectors, 34-36
Astroglia
   expression of type II glucocorticoid
      receptor, 130
   maturation and differentiation
      in primary culture, 127
Axotomy-induced retrograde degeneration, 85

Bad
   apoptotic action, 23
Basic fibroblast growth factor (bFGF)
   expression of IGF-I receptor, 25
   mitogenic action, 127
   neuroprotective action, 102
Bax
   apoptotic action, 23
Bcl-2
   anti-apoptopic action, 22-23
   expression in CNS and PNS, 35

Bcl-X$_l$
   anti-apoptotic action, 22-23
Bcl-Xs
   apoptotic action, 23
BDNF, see Brain derived neurotrophic factor
Brain derived neurotropic factor (BDNF)
   action on GSA production, 67

Canary
   expression of IGF-II in songnuclei, 6-8
Cerebellar granule cells (CGsC)
   apoptosis and necrosis, 60
   energetic state, 62
   survival, 62-64
Cerebrospinal fluid (CSF)
   IGF-I concentrations, 29
Choline-acetyltransferase (ChAT)
   saporin-induced hippocampal deple-
      tion, 54
Cholinergic pathways
   basal forebrain, 54
Ciliary neurotrophic factor (CNTF), 105
Cytokines
   apoptotic mechanisms, 17
   as mediators of IGF induction, 57

Demyelinating diseases
   prospects for therapy, 76
Des (1-3) IGF-I
   neuroprotection in brain injury, 100, 145
Diabetes
   neuropathy, 151
      IGF-I expression in sural nerves
         151-154
      involvement of growth factors, 154
Duchenne muscular distrophy (DMD)
   effect of IGF-I treatment, 123

EGF, see Epidermal growth factor
Epidermal growth factor
    anti-apoptotic activity, 57
    neurotropic activity, 127

Glucocorticoids
    interactions with IGF-I and bFGF, 130
    type II receptor in glial cells, 130
Glutamate
    excitotoxicity, 111
    receptors, 70
    sensitizing activity (GSA), 61, 66, 67
    transporter gene knock-out
        effects of IGF-I, 111
Glutamate-sensitizing activity (GSA)
    role of IGF-I, 64-68
Glycine-proline-glutamate (GPE)
    biological actions, 145
    effect on hypoxic-ischemic injury, 101
    pretreatment of hippocampal cultures
        146-148

High vocal center (HVC)
    expression of IGF-II, 7, 9
    neural afferents, 6
Hippocampus
    age induced deafferentation, 53
    expression of IGF-I, type I IGFR and
        IGFBPs, 48

IGF-I
    anti-apoptotic action, 17, 36, 61
        underlying mechanisms, 18-22
    antibodies
        effect on locomotion and passive
            avoidance, 135, 141
    as a neuronal rescue agent, 93, 94
        transport and cellular location, 95
    cerebrospinal fluid, 29
    CNS distribution, 28
    deficiency in humans, 3
    effects on ADP-ribosylation, 127
    expression in glial cells, 74
    gene expression
        correlation with age, 50-53
        developmental pattern, 28
    glutamate sensitivity, 64-68
    interactions with hormones and growth
        factor, 56, 127
    neuronal motility, 30-33

    neurotrophic properties, 28, 38
    NMDA-induced damage, 147, 148
    promotion of myelination, 73, 76
    receptor
        distribution, 105, 29
        expression in apoptosis, 25
        expression in sural nerves, 151, 154
        signaling pathways, 18-22
        distribution, 105, 29
    recovery of motor function, 109
    regulation of oligodendrocyte develop-
        ment, 72, 29
        signal transduction mechanisms, 76
    role in aging hippocampus, 56
    survival and neurite outgrowth, 33, 106
    transgenic models, 1-3, 29, 56 111
    treatment
        demyelinating diseases, 76
        models of motor neuron disease, 85,
            108
        neuromuscular disorders, 115-124
    trophic function in neuronal replace-
        ment, 5
IGF-II
    in choroid plexus and leptomenigeae, 9, 97
    induction by brain injury, 93
    knockout mice, 10
    regulation of neuronal plasticity, 8
    role in the adult brain, 10
    secretion into CSF, 9
    specific expression in HVC,RA, 7
IGFBP-1
    overexpression in Tg mice, 10
        developmental defects, 11
IGFBP-2
    expression in brain, 93
    induction following injury, 95
    role in oligodendrocyte regeneration, 75
IGFBP-3
    induction following injury, 93
IGFBP-4
    effect on motor neuron sprouting, 109
IGFBP-5
    induction following injury, 93
Insulin-like growth hormone binding pro-
    teins (IGFBPs) (see also individual com-
    ponents)
    role in modulating IGF action, 75
Insulin-receptor substrate-I (IRS-I)
    effect of IGF-I, 29

Interleukin-1β converting enzyme (ICE)
early PCD, 36
proteases
anti-apoptotic action, 23

Kainate receptors, 60

LH-RH
neuronal cell line, 127
L-Nitro-L-arginine methylester (NAME), 67

MAP kinase pathway
anti-apoptotic action of IGF-I, 18-21
Mnd mouse, 85
Motor neuron
axotomy-induced retrograde degeneration, 85
disease, 105, 106, 111
sprouting by botulinum toxin, 109
effect of IGF-I and GAGs, 86-93
Motor neuron disease, see also Amyotrophic lateral sclerosis
experimental models, 85
effect of IGF-I and GAGs, 86-93
rationale for IGF-I use, 105
survival in vitro and in vivo, 108
effect of IGF-I, 108
Multiple sclerosis
demyelination, 72
IGF-I therapeutic potential, 76
MyD, see Myotonic dystrophy
Myotonic dystrophy
effect of IGF-I treatment, 121-123

NGF, see Nerve growth factor
Nerve growth factor (NGF)
differentiation of PC12 cells, 18
Neuromuscular disorders (see also individual diseases)
treatment with IGF-I, 115
Neurotropic factors (NTFs) (see also individual factors)
interactions with IGF-I, 56
intercellular signalling agents, 127
Nitric oxide synthase
effect of GPE on asphyxia-induced loss, 101

N-methyl-D-aspartate (NMDA)
induced cell damage, 148
effect of receptor antagonist, 147
NMDA, see N-methyl-D-aspartate
N-methyl-D-aspartate
antagonists, 146
damage of hippocampal cultures, 146-148
receptors
GSA-induced up-regulation, 67

Olfactory bulb (OB)
cytoarchitecture, 4
IGF-I sensitivity, 4
mitral cells, 4
Oligodendrocytes
development, 72, 76
expression of IGFBPs, 75
Open field testing, 138

Passive avoidance testing, 137
Peripheral nervous system (PNS)
IGF-I expression, 105
myelin formation by Schwann cells, 72
PI3'-Kinase pathway
anti-apoptotic action of IGF-I, 18-21
Post-polio syndrome (PPS)
effect of IGF-I treatment, 115, 120
Programmed cell death (PCD), see Apoptosis

Rat cerebellar granule cells (CGCs)
apopotosis and cell death, 47
Reactive oxygen species (ROS)
scavengers
inhibition of apoptosis, 64
Retention phase, 138
ROS, see Reactive oxygen species

Tumor necrosis factor (TNF), 17, 67

Ultrasonic vocalization, 137

Wobbler mouse
effect of IGF-I and GAGs treatment, 86-88
model of motor neuron disease, 85

Zebra finch
expression of IGF-I in songnuclei, 6